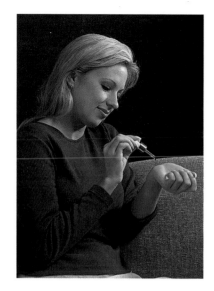
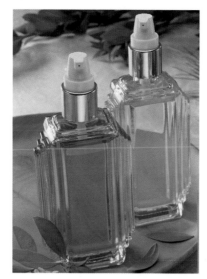
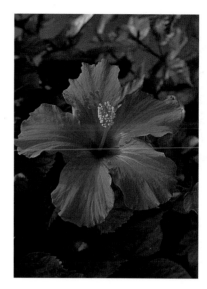

Aromatherapy
Basics

David Schiller
& Carol Schiller

Photography by
Marvin & Lynne Carlton

® Sterling Publishing Co.,

**Library of Congress
Cataloging-in-Publication Data**

Schiller, Carol.
  Aromatherapy basics / Carol Schiller & David Schiller : photography by Marvin & Lynne Carlton.
       p. cm.
  Includes index.
  ISBN 0-8069-9785-0
  1. Aromatherapy. I. Schiller, David, 1942–   II. Title. RM666.A68S3523 1998
615'.321—dc21   98-7678
                                            CIP

10 9 8 7 6 5 4 3 2 1

Published by Sterling Publishing Company, Inc. 387 Park Avenue South, New York, N.Y. 10016

© 1998 by David Schiller and Carol Schiller

Distributed in Canada by Sterling Publishing c/o Canadian Manda Group, One Atlantic Avenue, Suite 105, Toronto, Ontario, Canada M6K 3E7

Distributed in Great Britain and Europe by Cassell PLC, Wellington House, 125 Strand, London WC2R 0BB, England

Distributed in Austrailia by Capricorn Link (Austrailia) Pty. Ltd., P.O. Box 6651, Baulkham Hills, Business Centre, NSW 2153, Austrailia

Printed in China
All rights reserved

Design by Laura Hammond Hough
Sterling ISBN 0-8069-9785-0

Acknowledgments

We would like to thank the following people and companies who graciously contributed their time, effort, and products for the making of this book:

- Charles Marchese of *ABA Packaging Corporation* in Holtsville, New York, for the beautiful glass bottles, droppers, lotion pumps, mist sprays, and accessories.
- Rosemarie Tavares-Silva of *Pochet of America* in Wayne, New Jersey, for the fancy and elegant perfume glass bottles and stoppers.
- Marcel Lavabre of *Aroma Vera Inc.*, in Los Angeles, California, for the aroma lamps, lightbulb rings, and diffuser.
- Brigette Pauli and Michelle Anderson of *AKO-ISMET Electrical Appliances, Inc.*, in Franklin, Tennessee, for the diffuser.
- *Caswell-Massey*, in Dover, Delaware, for the classical fragrance lamp.
- Michael Sopkiw of *Miron Glass USA*, in Los Angeles, California, for the violet glass bottles.
- Models appearing in the book: Kim Boat, Shelena Bohling, Amie Coleman, Jeffrey Schiller, Aztechan Lee Fuller, Carol Schiller, and David Schiller.
- Marvin and Lynne Carlton for their great photography work.
- Steven and Cherylanne for the use of their beautiful home.
- Vivian Bitahy for her hairstyling.
- Roslyn Blumenthal for her valuable insight.
- The staff and librarians at the Glendale Public Library in Glendale, Arizona.
- The people at Sterling Publishing Company: Sheila Anne Barry, Acquisitions Director, for her creative ingenuity that contributed to the conception and many ideas that enhanced this book; Hazel Chan, our Editor, for her outstanding efforts; John Woodside, Editorial Director; Charles Nurnberg, Executive Vice President; and Nalini Ramjit, Publicist.

Dedicated to all people who treasure,
cherish, and live in peace and harmony with nature.
For it is they who can experience the great joy
and deep inner fulfillment from the
close connection with our precious earth.

A fragrant scent wafting through the air
seemingly appearing insignificant —
yet having the power to evoke feelings and emotions;
and produce memories that can last for the duration of a lifetime.

DAVID SCHILLER

Contents

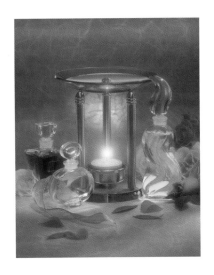

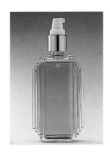

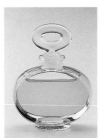

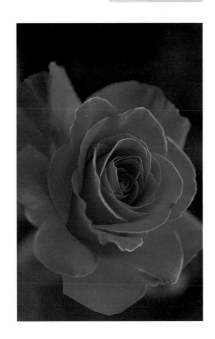

5

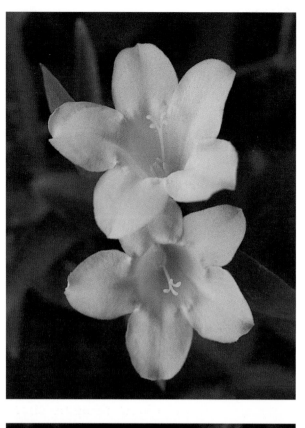
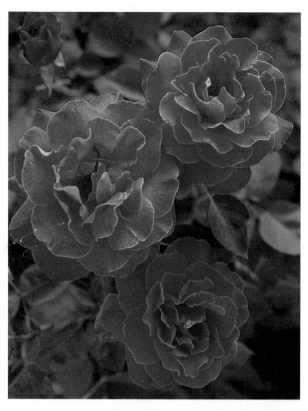
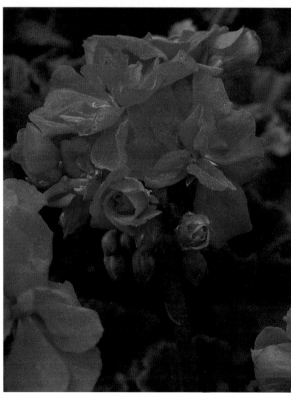
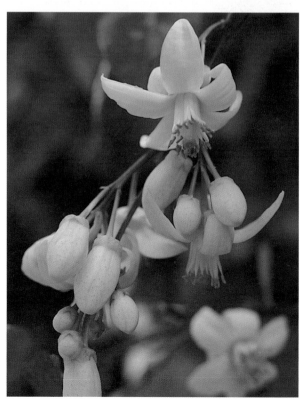

Introduction
Our Precious Gift from Nature

The sweet hypnotic scent of a sunny citrus grove in full bloom bringing cheer and joy to the heart. The sensual fragrance from the flowers of the ylang-ylang tree producing a feeling of euphoric sensation. The herbs, trees, and shrubs growing in the wild along a countryside road generously broadcasting their uplifting scents after a rain shower. The dazzling display of colorful flowers with their petals fluttering in the passing summer breeze inviting all to smell their delightful perfume.

The magnificent fragrances and extraordinary beauty of nature's aromatic plants are unsurpassable. They enrich our life, bring us joy, embellish our surroundings, lift our spirit in time of illness, give us solace, comfort, and condolence during times of grieving, and heighten the festivity of every important celebration.

Aromatic plants have existed on the earth long before humans. Some plants are believed to have been here for over 100 million years. Fossils have been found containing roses at least 20–30 million years old.

Aromatic plants have played an important role in the turn of events in history. Wars were fought to gain their possession, new lands were discovered in search for them, and cities that traded these valuable commodities became powerful centers of commerce. Some of the fragrant resins and oils were in such great demand they commanded prices comparable to, or even higher than, gold, silver, and precious jewels.

The ancient Sumerians, Assyrians, and Egyptians bathed in waters fragrantly scented with aromatic oils. Assyrian women were well-known in the Middle East for their beautiful and silky smooth complexions. They used skin lotions made from a mixture of oils and resins of frankincense, cypress, and cedarwood.

The ancient Egyptians were so enthralled with the various aromatic scents that they applied a different fragrance to each part of their body. Some of the upper-class men wore up to sixteen different fragrances in one day. The women scented their hair and colored their skin and nails with a dye made from henna. Foods were scented and flavored, flower blossoms were strewn throughout households, statues were crowned with fragrant wreaths, and incense was burned in the streets during festivals. When high-ranking dignitaries died, they were embalmed with aromatics, and aromatics were placed in their tombs with fragrances to accompany them into the afterworld.

The ancient Egyptian priests were the perfumers, healers, and first-known large-scale producers of aromatic essences. They produced the resins and oils in a laboratory that was located in every Egyptian temple, then blended the fragrant materials for their own use as well as for the kings, queens, wealthy individuals, and other prominent people of the temples and governments.

During religious services, fragrant waters were used in the anointing rituals, and incense was burned to protect against evil spirits and make prayers more effective. It was believed that smoke from the burning incense created heavenly pathways through which prayers traveled to reach the Gods. The intoxicating fumes also helped the worshippers enter into a euphoric state. Concoctions were made of the various highly prized fragrant resins and oils: cedarwood, myrrh, frankincense, cassia, cinnamon, mint, juniper, spikenard, saffron, galbanum, and henna.

Not only did the ancient Greeks emulate the Egyptian uses of aromatics; they also added their own extravagance. Incense was burned daily in the homes of the wealthy as well as at celebrations, funerals, and religious services. Physicians treated illnesses with fragrant oils and ointments. Athletes and soldiers anointed themselves to gain courage and strength. Victorious heroes from athletic games and military battles were honored by being crowned with aromatic garlands.

The ancient Romans took full advantage of the many uses of aromatics. They doused their bodies extensively with perfume, and scented furniture, clothing, the water in the fountains, and even their large amphitheaters. Men visited barbershops daily to be shaven, then had their faces massaged with scented oils. Perfume shops served as popular meeting places and perfumers became as socially respected as doctors and apothecaries.

Soldiers scented their bodies and hair as well as their weapons and military banners. At celebrations, heroic army commanders were presented with fragrant crowns to wear, but the ultimate award of honor was the crown made of laurel leaves given to the victorious generals during the triumphal celebration.

The royal Roman banquets were quite lavish and were the epitome of aromatic extravagance. Attendees at the feasts had their hands and feet washed with scented waters. Rose crowns were placed on their heads and rose garlands around their necks. Birds were drenched with fragrance and released to fly overhead in the rooms where the people congregated. Wine, scented with fragrance, was drunk and sprayed on the guests. Aromatic fragrances spewed out of silver pipes above the rooms. At one of Emperor Nero's great festivities a guest was asphyxiated from the heavy vapors given off from the showers of roses.

By the 1st century, Rome became the bathing capital of the world. There were about one thousand bathhouses located throughout the city—the large ones having the capacity to accommodate up to two thousand bathers at a time. People came to bathe, socialize, and, afterward, receive a pleasurable massage with fragrant oils and unguents.

Over time there was a decline in the morality of the bathers, and promiscuity leading to lewd and lascivious acts became commonplace. During the reign of Hadrian in the 2nd century, the bathing together of both genders was outlawed and the time periods of bathhouse use for men and women were alternated.

Nero bathed in water fragranced with rose wine and slept on a bed full of rose petals. At his wife's funeral, a greater amount of aromatics was used than what Arabia produced in an entire year. Nero's prolific use of aromatics caused the Roman government's treasury to go bankrupt. The absurdity of the wasteful use of aromatics reached even a higher point when, in later times, the Roman emperors ordered the general populace to burn incense daily to honor and worship them.

Overindulgence of fragrances by the masses infuriated the Church. Perfume use became associated with sin and degeneracy, and the Church condemned the personal use of aromatics. Consequently, the widespread use of fragrant resins and oils came to an abrupt halt in Europe. However, plant oil use still continued in the Middle and Far East.

In China, incense was burned to honor ancestors and past emperors. The Chinese people were fond of jasmine flowers. Gardens extending for miles were solely devoted to growing jasmine. The ladies wore the flowers in their hair during the day. In the evening, they wore head garlands and rubbed the fragrance on their body. At night, they hung the flowers over their bed. Teas and wines flavored with jasmine flowers were also quite popular.

Aromatics also played an important role in India's culture. Sandalwood, jasmine, rose, and champaca flowers were popularly used. In the Hindu religion, sandalwood oil was incorporated into religious, wedding, and funeral services. During worship services, perfumed water was applied to the body with the belief that it was purifying.

In the 14th century, the Black Plague raged through Europe and Asia, taking an estimated toll of 75 million lives. The resins and oils of cedar, clove, pine, sage, rosemary, and thyme were burned in the streets, hospitals, and sickrooms in a desperate attempt to fight off the deadly infectious organisms. In 1665, many lives were lost from another plague that broke out in Europe. Again, aromatic substances were burned to disinfect everything against the deadly bacterial onslaught. It is said that perfumers and individuals who handled and used aromatics, as well as those who lived in towns where the aromatic plants were extensively grown, were virtually immune to the ravages of the plague and survived.

Aromatics were popular in England during the reign of Queen Elizabeth I. Fragrant plants were used to scent linens, and pillows and mattresses were stuffed with calming fragrances to promote a good night's sleep. Sachets containing dried leaves and flower petals were hung on chairs, furniture, and bedposts. Lavender, melissa, mint, basil, chamomile, sage, hyssop, and thyme were placed around the home and on the floor to provide a fresh indoor scent. They were also planted in window boxes and gardens. Scented waters were popular as well as gloves that were impregnated with fragrances.

In the mid-19th century, scientists began producing synthetic versions of the essential oils, replacing these precious natural substances that had been treasured since the beginning of time. Methyl salicylate oil was artificially produced to substitute for natural wintergreen and sweet birch oil. A synthetic version of coumarin replaced natural coumarin; benzyl chloride was used in place of bitter almond; vanillin was used for vanilla; and ionone became the synthetic version of violet oil.

Synthetic fragrances are usually produced from petroleum derivatives. They not only pose harmful side effects for the individuals using them, but processing these chemicals also pollutes the environment. Essential oils, on the other hand, are natural and are in perfect harmony with the earth.

Today, more people are realizing that the continued use of harmful synthetic chemicals has produced many far-reaching ill-effects. Not only has the environment undergone devastating damage, but the number of individuals suffering from debilitating environmental illnesses has been steadily increasing. It has become self-evident that we must return to a more natural lifestyle and replace the deleterious chemicals in our daily life with beneficial plant products derived from nature. We must do all we can to improve our situation.

Incorporate the aromatic oils into your everyday life and experience their positive impact. Enliven, elate, gladden, rejoice, and cheer. Refresh, revive, renew, rejuvenate, regenerate, invigorate, stimulate, energize, excite, heighten, and arouse. Calm, still, quiet, soothe, and relax. Feel special and privileged. Take advantage of each opportunity to enjoy life more. Treasure each moment and be thankful for the extraordinary gift nature has given us—the precious essential oils.

Chapter 1
What Is Aromatherapy?

In the past, when you've smelled an aroma, you've most likely only judged it from a standpoint of whether you liked it or not. Now you will learn to go far beyond that point by focusing primarily on how the oil affects you, rather than liking or disliking it. Chances are you will find most of the oils to your liking. However, some of the oils that you initially dislike may eventually become among your favorites after you've used them and experienced their wonderfully remarkable benefits.

The following is a scene in our aromatherapy class. These classes provide a chance for people to learn about and experience the incredible properties of the essential oils and use them to enrich their lives.

Sheila volunteered to experience the oils in front of the class and share her input. As she made herself comfortable in the chair next to me, I instructed her to close her eyes and take a few deep breaths to help settle her mind and become relaxed. Within a few moments, she visibly became more calm and at ease. She was now ready to begin.

"I am going to give you three essential oils to individually sniff. With each one, I want you to pay close attention to, and become aware of, any effects you may experience as you smell each aroma. Take your time and be patient with yourself, since it can take a few minutes to pinpoint and articulate the effects."

I uncap the bottle of essential oil and hand it to Sheila. "Hold the bottle about an inch underneath your nose. . . . Take slow deep breaths and avoid exhaling into the bottle."

Sheila brings the bottle up to her nose and, upon taking a few sniffs, she immediately smiles and says, "This aroma is nice and sweet. . . . It smells familiar. . . . vanilla!" As she sniffs more, she continues, "It makes me feel happy."

"Do you feel any physical changes?"

Sheila takes a moment to become aware of her body by moving her head side to side and rotating her shoulders. "Yes. . . . I feel less tension in my neck and shoulders. . . . I tend to store stress in these areas." In a lower tone of voice she continues, "I feel more calm and settled. . . . peaceful. . . . I like this feeling."

"Excellent Sheila, you're correct. This is vanilla oil. It's a good oil to calm, reduce stress, and uplift the mood. . . . But this vanilla is CO_2 extracted and is different from the common type of vanilla extract that is sold in grocery stores. The CO_2 vanilla is purer and of higher quality, containing no alcohol or additives. We only use the CO_2 extract in our classes. Now let's go on to the next oil, which is cinnamon leaf."

Sheila takes the bottle from me and inhales the aroma several times. "Mm. . . . this aroma is warm. . . . It reminds me of when I'd walk into my grandmother's house on a cold winter's day while she was baking cinnamon cookies. I felt such warm, loving feelings and closeness." She puts down the bottle and continues. "I really miss those days."

"It's a common occurrence for the scent of the oils to evoke memories. I'm glad the cinnamon oil was able to help you bring back this fond memory. What else are you feeling?"

"I feel warm and comforted," she says, looking content.

"Very good. Now let's try the last oil."

Immediately as Sheila sniffs the bottle she becomes wide awake and springs up in her chair. "Wow! This aroma is much stronger than the others. It smells like one of my favorite chewing gum flavors. This is peppermint oil, isn't it?"

"Yes," I reply.

Sheila inhales the oil a few more times and excitedly says, "These vapors really travel deep into my sinuses and breathing. I am alert. . . . clear-headed. This is great! It's so exciting to experience each oil, I can't wait to try the others!"

What Are Essential Oils?

Aromatherapy is the use of pure essential oils extracted from grasses, flower petals, seeds, fruit rinds, buds, resins, bark, wood, twigs, stems, leaves, roots, or rhizomes. Essential oils are responsible for the fragrance emitted by plants. These oils vary in color, are insoluble in water at room temperature, and have a watery consistency except for resins, some florals, and others such as patchouli, which tend to be heavier in viscosity.

Essential oils are quite different from carrier oils. They are highly volatile and evaporate rapidly when exposed to air. Carrier oils, also known as vegetal oils, are extracted from nuts, seeds, fruits, and vegetables. They are made up of fatty acids, which give the oils a greasy texture. Carrier oils are used to dilute essential oils in massage oil blends as well as blends for skin and hair care, protecting the skin from possible irritation by the concentrated essential oils. Unlike essential oils, carrier oils are not as stable and have a shorter shelf life.

We may not realize it but practically everyone is in contact with essential oils on many occasions each day. The oils are ingredients in toothpastes, chewing gum, candy, soft drinks, food flavorings, household products, cosmetics, perfumes, aftershave lotions, colognes, soaps, skin and hair care products, and personal hygiene products. According to William Poundstone in the book *Big Secrets*, the secret formula for Coca-Cola includes the essential oils of nutmeg, cassia, lemon, orange, lime, neroli, lavender, and coriander.

The essential oil may be concentrated in a specific part of a plant or spread out in several areas. For example, the orange tree yields oil from its flower blossoms, leaves, twigs, and rind of the fruit. The clove tree contains oil in the buds, stems, and leaves. The whole plant of peppermint, lemongrass, and gingergrass is used, whereas oil is extracted only from the flowers of rose, jasmine, helichrysum, and ylang-ylang.

Some essential oils are obtained from dried plant materials like pimento berries and clove buds; others are from fresh materials like neroli flowers, litsea cubeba berries, and the leaves of the eucalyptus citriodora tree. Some oils are extracted from ripe berries, such as juniper berries and litsea cubeba; and others are extracted from unripe berries, such as black pepper and pimento berry.

The quality and quantity of an essential oil produced from a plant depends on several factors: where the plant is grown, altitude, moisture, climate, condition of the soil, season, the time of day or night the plant material is harvested, and the extraction process. The ylang-ylang tree bears flowers year-round, but the months in which the flowers contain the highest yield of oil are May and June. Roses are picked early in the morning before sunrise; jasmine flowers are picked at dusk before they are a day old.

Methods of Extraction

The extraction process helps to determine the purity of an oil. It is important to be knowledgeable about the different methods of extraction before purchasing carrier and essential oils.

STEAM DISTILLATION: Steam from boiling water is used to release the essential oils from the plant material. The steam is then cooled and condensed into a liquid. The oil separates and floats on top of the water, where it is skimmed off. This extraction method is most extensively used and produces a good-quality essential oil.

CARBON DIOXIDE GAS EXTRACTION: There are two extraction processes in this method. One is called Select, the other is Total. In the Select method, the oil is extracted at a temperature of around 87.8°F (31°C). The plant material is placed in a chamber and then the compressed CO_2 gas is released. As the gas passes through the plant material, it takes the components into solution. When the process is completed the pressure is lowered, and the extracted components precipitate out and are collected. The CO_2 gas is then recompressed and recycled to be used again without leaving any residues in the extracted oil. The extracted oil contains selected components similar to the oils that are steam distilled. In the Total extracted method, the plant material is processed at a higher temperature. The extracted oil from this method contains more components than from the Select method.

Since the CO_2 process equipment is extremely costly, the essential oils produced are more expensive.

EXPELLER, MECHANICALLY, OR COLD PRESSED: Seeds, nuts, vegetables, fruits, and fruit peels are pressed without the use of high heat. This is an excellent method to produce a quality oil. However, large amounts of these oils are usually refined afterward using high heat and harsh chemicals. Therefore, it is important to check the label on the container in order to ensure that the oil is unrefined so that it contains all the valuable nutrients.

MACERATION: Flowers are soaked in hot oil until their cells rupture and the oil absorbs the essence.

SOLVENT EXTRACTION: The plant material is bathed in solvents such as hexane and other toxic chemicals that extract the oil. This method is less costly and extracts a greater amount of oil. However, toxic residues remain in the oil, which makes this product undesirable for aromatherapy use. Absolute flower oils and a high percentage of vegetable oils are extracted in this manner.

REFINING PROCESS FOR VEGETAL/CARRIER OILS: After the oil has been extracted from the plant material, it is usually put through a refining process that includes these steps:

Examples of Specific Parts of Plants Used to Produce Each Essential Oil

❧

ESSENTIAL OILS	PART OF PLANT THE OIL IS EXTRACTED FROM
Gingergrass	Grass
Champaca Flower, Helichrysum, Jasmine, Neroli, Rose, Ylang-Ylang	Flowers
Chamomile, Clary Sage, Lavender, Marjoram	Flowering Tops
Spikenard	Roots
Amyris, Cabreuva, Cedarwood, Guaiacwood, Sandalwood	Wood Chips
Eucalyptus Citriodora, Patchouli, Ravensara Aromatica, Sage	Leaves
Grapefruit, Lemon, Lime, Mandarin, Orange, Tangerine	Peel of the Fruit
Copaiba	Resin
Juniper Berry, Litsea Cubeba, Pimento Berry	Berries
Ambrette Seed, Fennel	Seeds

Degumming: Removes chlorophyll, vitamins, and minerals from the oil.
Refining: An alkaline solution called lye is added to refine the oil.
Bleaching: Fuller's earth is added as a bleaching agent and then filtered out to further remove nutritive substances. The oil in this state becomes clear.
Deodorizing: The oil is deodorized by steam distillation at high temperatures over 450°F (232°C) for 30–60 minutes.
Winterizing: The oil is then cooled and filtered. This process prevents the oil from becoming cloudy during cold temperatures. The finished product is nutrient-deficient, with only fatty acids remaining.

Synthetic vs. Natural

Prior to the isolation of individual components of essential oils and the production of synthetic fragrances in the 19th century, the smell of an essence was representative of the plant material it originally came from. In today's synthetic fragrances, the true natural substances are mostly absent. The scent of a bouquet of flowers may not even contain one molecule of the essence of a real flower, or a food containing the flavoring of vanilla may smell and taste like vanilla, but yet it may not contain a drop of real vanilla.

Chemists are greatly skilled in their ability to cheaply produce synthetic versions of fragrances similar in scent to those of the expensive essences. The purpose of their work is to create fragrant compounds to scent products and perfumes so that they are more appealing for purchase. However, these synthetic chemicals, based on their value, are no match in comparison to the natural essential oils.

The synthetic compounds not only don't contain the beneficial properties of plants, but they can be irritating to the skin, respiratory system, and nervous system as well. The processing of these chemicals also pollutes the earth, water, and air. Essential oils, on the other hand, are much more than just a fragrance; they are the life force of the plants that they are extracted from. These precious essences work on a much deeper level, affecting us not only on the physical but on the mental and spiritual level as well. They help balance our body, improve our well-being, and put us into greater harmony with the natural world. They protect us with their antibacterial properties, reduce our stress, and give us comfort, reassurance, and pleasure.

How to Select and Purchase Pure Oils

It is unfortunate, but a high percentage of oils that are commonly sold to the public are adulterated. This is done in order to increase profits without much concern for the consequences to the consumers. Some of the adulteration can be comprised of adding a cheaper oil to a more

ESSENTIAL OIL	COMMONLY ADULTERATED WITH
Bergamot	Lime
Cinnamon Bark	Cinnamon Leaf, Clove Leaf
Fennel (Sweet)	Fennel (Bitter)
Geranium	Citronella, Palmarosa
Jasmine	Ylang-Ylang
Juniper Berry	Juniper wood and twigs
Lavender	Lavandin
Lemon	Orange
Neroli	Orange, Petitgrain
Pimento Berry	Clove
Rose	Palmarosa
Rosemary	Eucalyptus
Patchouli	Cedarwood, Copaiba, Gurjun Balsam
Peppermint	Cornmint
Sandalwood	Amyris, Cedarwood, Copaiba
Ylang-Ylang	Cananga

expensive oil in order to "stretch" it. Many other more serious adulterations take place by adding synthetic as well as fractionalized components, which contaminate the oils. This practice is common knowledge in the essential oil industry and referred to as "making a soup." Each time the oil changes hands, the possibility increases for the original oil to become more contaminated with adulterants.

Substantial variations exist in the difference of prices the various essential oils sell for. The determining factors are:

1. The labor intensity required to harvest the plant.
2. The extraction method used.
3. The yield of oil per plant.
4. The supply and demand of the particular plant material at a given time.

For example: In order to produce 1 pound of rose oil, over 4,000 pounds (1,800 kilograms) of roses must be picked and processed, whereas 1 pound (½ kilogram) of lavender oil requires only about 250 pounds (112½ kilograms) of lavender flowers.

The charts on the following page group the essential and carrier oils according to their purchase cost.

The highest-grade and most effective oils are produced from plants that are grown wild and away from polluted sources, or are cultivated by natural farming methods without the use of chemical pesticides, herbicides, or any other unnatural substances. It is important to select carrier oils that are expeller, mechanically, or cold pressed and unrefined, and essential oils that have been CO_2 extracted, steam distilled, or, in the case of citrus fruit oils, cold pressed.

Retail oils are generally packaged in five different categories:

1. *Essential oils* are individual pure essential oils with nothing added.
2. *Carrier oils* can be found in a health food store in the vegetable oil section.
3. *Oil blends* can either be a single essential oil mixed in a carrier oil or several different essential oils mixed in a carrier oil.
4. *Fragrance oils* are generally synthetic chemicals mixed together.
5. *Skin care oils* are a blend of carrier oils, with or without essential oils, and can contain synthetic chemicals.

Investigating to find pure, high-quality oil is quite a learning experience and it requires comparing the same oil of different brands with one another. Contacting the company and speaking with the appropriate person who oversees the purchasing of oils can help gain insight into the philosophy and integrity of the company.

Essential Oils

◉

LEAST EXPENSIVE	MODERATELY EXPENSIVE	MORE EXPENSIVE
Cassia Bark	Amyris	Ambrette Seed
Cedarwood (Atlas)	Cabreuva	Chamomile (Roman)
Cinnamon Leaf	Clary Sage	Champaca Flower
Clove Bud	Cypress	Helichrysum
Copaiba	Fir Needle	Hyssop Decumbens
Eucalyptus Citriodora	Geranium	Juniper Berry
Fennel (Sweet)	Gingergrass	Manuka
Grapefruit	Guaiacwood	Myrtle
Lemon	Havozo Bark	Neroli
Lime	Lavender	Rose
Litsea Cubeba	Mandarin	Sandalwood
Orange	Marjoram	Spikenard
Peppermint	Patchouli	Vanilla
Rosemary	Pimento Berry	Ylang-Ylang
Sage (Spanish)	Ravensara Aromatica	
Spearmint	Spruce	
Tangerine	Thyme	

Carrier Oils

◉

LEAST EXPENSIVE	MODERATELY EXPENSIVE	MORE EXPENSIVE
Almond (Sweet)	Carrot Root (Heliocarrot)	Borage
Avocado	Kukui Nut	Calophyllum (Tamanu)
Cocoa Butter	Sisymbrium	Evening Primrose
Grapeseed		Pine Nut
Jojoba		Sea Buckthorn Berry
Macadamia Nut		
Pistachio Nut		
Sesame		
Shea Butter		

Chapter 2
Why We Need Aromatherapy

Years ago, before the world became so industrialized, people had a close relationship with one another as well as with the natural environment. Life was tough but members in a family worked closely together and helped one another to better increase the chances of survival. People lived in communities of small farms surrounded by wild plants, bushes, shrubs, and forest land. The air was fresh and crisp. There were rivers, lakes, running streams, and springs nearby providing a source of fresh clean water to drink and bathe in. Those who planted had a deep understanding of caring for the soil as well as nurturing and enriching the earth to ensure healthy crops year after year.

Today, the vast majority of people live in cities. A large number of people live alone and families are fragmented, more than half are single-parent families, and even the families that are together—in many of them the members have little interaction with one another and lack the closeness and support system of the traditional family lifestyle of the past.

In the large cities, the air is polluted. At times, it gets so bad that some cities issue notices advising a certain portion of the population to stay indoors, since breathing the outdoor air will worsen their condition. Filtering devices are placed on faucets and shower heads to reduce the toxicity of water for drinking or taking a shower. The sounds of nature are nearly nonexistent, and the little there are, are drowned out by the sounds of automobiles, buses, trucks, ear-piercing emergency vehicle sirens, blasting jackhammers, and other demolition and construction noises. There are violent crimes, burglaries, and suicides, and the courts that handle domestic family conflicts can't keep up with the large volume of cases. It is certainly difficult for people to function in a healthy way in such an environment.

As ailments caused by stress and pollution continue to rise each year, more people are turning to nature's herbs and essential oils to help them better cope with life in the city. Essential oils are the vital life force of the plants from which they are extracted. They play an invaluable role in reconnecting us to the natural world on which we desperately depend for well-being and helping us get closer to the people we care for.

The formulas in this book offer a large selection to choose from. Mist and diffuse delightful aromas into the air to resemble the fragrances of a sweet flower garden, a clean fresh uplifting citrus grove, or the refreshing, reviving scents of a patch of peppermint and spearmint plants.

Prepare your own deodorants, bath oils, breath fresheners, and body powders to stay fresh all day. Revitalize your skin and hair to look younger and more beautiful. Enjoy a candlelight dinner in a delightful aromatic setting and afterward take pleasure in giving and receiving a romantic massage.

Unlock your mind and allow the greatness within you to develop more each day. Improve your life with the *Be the Best You Can Be*, *Recognize Your Treasures*, *Think Positive Thoughts*, *Make a Difference*, and *Wake Up to a Great Day!* formulas. Improve the way you convey your feelings to the people around you with *Express Appreciation* and *Communicate Effectively*. Experience an inner feeling of contentment with *Peace and Calm*. Spend quality time with someone special with *Get Closer to the Ones You Love*. Reach new heights of accomplishment with *Stop Procrastination* and *Laziness Relief*, and enjoy life to the fullest with *Open Your Heart for Love*, *Choose To Be Happy*, *Practice Kindness*, and *Savor These Precious Moments*. Encourage better recall of your dreams with the *Dream* formulas and gain insight to the valuable information and messages provided by your subconscious mind.

On occasion, people who have used the dream formulas have experienced precognitive dreams. A young lady in her 20's, who was planning to get married in a few months, was taking our aromatherapy classes. She was working on her homework assignment and selected to use a dream formula. She applied the oils before going to sleep and later that night she had a dream that her fiancé was looking for her with the intention to seriously harm her. She hid underneath her bed hoping he would not find her. When she awoke, she shrugged off what she dreamt and considered it to be just a bad dream.

When she presented the results of her homework assignment at the next class, she shared the details of the dream. She was then asked if her fiancé had previously shown any tendencies toward violent behaviors and if she had any reservations about getting married. She replied how wonderful a person he was and that she was looking forward to the wedding.

Two years later, she divorced her husband on the grounds of physical abuse and the possible endangerment she felt for her life; he had threatened to kill her if she ever left him.

Another student used the dream formula and dreamt she came early to a party and read the list of all the guests who were invited. Two days later, she returned home from work, not knowing that her mother had arranged a surprise party for her and invited her friends and classmates she knew from years ago. The people who were present were the same people whose names appeared on the guest list in her dream.

On the humorous side, one of our students in his 30's walked out of an all-day aromatherapy workshop feeling and smelling great from the uplifting oils that were used on him during the class. Afterward he got together with a group of friends for a social gathering. At the gathering, someone from behind reached out and grabbed him by the back of his shirt, pulled him close, then came around and hugged and squeezed him. To his surprise, it was a woman he had known for a number of years; this was the first time she had ever demonstrated this type of behavior. At the next class he spoke about this episode and expressed how flattered he was. He credited the aromas from the essential oils for being responsible for this incident.

It doesn't take long for people who use the oils regularly to recognize their great value and respect their ability to perform effectively, not only on a physical level, but on an emotional and spiritual level also. Even though the oils cannot completely replace our inherent need to interact with the natural environment, we can still derive enormous benefits from their use. And they can help to relieve the unnatural lifestyle of city life that severely lacks the beauty and health benefits of trees, flowers, and other plants.

Chapter 3
How to Use Aromatherapy

The Importance of Our Sense of Smell

Recognizing her scent, a month-old infant cuddles up to its mother's breast, knowing she is the source for nourishment, love, and comfort. A burning odor coming from the kitchen alerts us to add water to the food cooking on the stove. The food on our dinner plate doesn't smell quite right, so we avoid eating it. Lucky for us, our nose analyzes all food and drink before they enter our mouth. We smell the aroma of food we really enjoy—all of a sudden our mouth waters, our appetite perks up, and we are in a better mood. The scent of a beautiful bouquet of flowers at a festive celebration gives us happy memories for the rest of our life.

Each time we inhale a breath of air, only about 2% of the aroma reaches the olfactory epithelium in our nose. The epithelium consists of two patches of tissue about the size of one square inch located in the upper rear of the nasal cavities. This is the area where we detect smell. The olfactory nerve contains about ten million smell receptors that protrude from mucous membranes. These receptors, in the form of hairs, collect the scent of vapors and convert them into signals that are transmitted first to the olfactory nerve, in the form of electrical impulses, and then to the olfactory bulb for processing in the limbic system.

The limbic system is made up of a collection of structures in the brain, such as the amygdala, hippocampus, and hypothalamus, that regulate the automatic body functions, behaviors, moods, emotions, sexual activity and reproduction, stress levels, appetite, learning ability, creativity, and long-term memory.

Scent signals can play an important part in provoking feelings and memories. The subconscious mind stores memories in a memory bank. Smelling a recognizable scent may trigger a response to the memories and emotions associated with it. The response generated can cause changes in body temperature, appetite, stress level, and sexual arousal.

For a substance to be smelled, certain characteristics must be present. The odor molecules must be volatile, or able to become airborne in a gaseous form. The vaporization has to occur for a long enough duration so that it won't dissipate before it is sensed. And the vapors need to have the ability to disperse; otherwise the odor remains faint since it is locked in a small fixed area.

The farther people become removed from the natural environment, the less they depend on smell for survival. We use our sense of smell to a far lesser extent than animals and insects. In nature, the major purpose of scent is to insure the survival of the species for current as well as future generations. Examples abound of the use of scent as a communication medium to convey vital information. Scents mark territorial boundaries, protect against danger, make a trail to find the way back home, and attract a partner for mating.

The keenness of the sense of smell is directly related to the amount of estrogen hormone in the body. Therefore, women in their childbearing years rate highest in olfactory sensitivity, since these are years when the estrogen levels are at their peak. Women are about one thousand times more sensitive to pheromone odors just before ovulation than at any other time during their cycle.

At the University of California, studies were conducted on the effects of scent on mothers and babies. Sixty percent of the 6-week-old infants could distinguish between the scent of their mother's breast and those of another mother. The mothers were blindfolded and given a choice of three babies 6 hours after giving birth. Sixty-one percent of the mothers correctly chose their own infant.

Scent association also plays a key role in consumer choices of which products they purchase. As a result, companies spend large sums of money each year on research to make products more appealing to the senses in order to increase sales.

Women shoppers were given three identical batches of nylon stockings to choose from. The first was the regular unscented, the second had a fruity scent, and the third was floral. The floral-scented hosiery was favored and judged to be the softest and of better quality.

When sales of shoes made with synthetic materials were doing poorly, a shoe company decided to fragrance them with a leather scent. As a result, their sales improved sharply.

Identical shoes were for sale in two rooms. One room was scented with a floral scent, while the other room was unscented. Out of the thirty-one participants in the study, twenty-six preferred the shoes in the scented room and were willing to pay a higher price for them.

In a test study, a shampoo was judged to be ineffective, but when only the fragrance was changed, the shampoo received the best rating.

The scent of pine was considered a favorite of women when it was used in cleaning products. But when the pine scent was used to fragrance facial tissues, the tissues were judged to be too rough.

Supermarkets and bakeries have known that when the scent of baked goods is wafted through the store, bakery product sales increase. That is where the phrase "They're selling like hot cakes" originally came from.

A study showed sales of popcorn doubled in movie theaters when the smell of buttered popcorn was diffused throughout the air.

An area in a gambling casino that was scented with a floral fragrance increased slot machine revenues by 45%.

A study conducted at Washington State University showed that customers are more likely to return to a store with a pleasant scent.

Even though our sense of smell is highly underrated in this modern society, unrealized to some, we still immensely depend upon it. It is important to treasure and fully appreciate this invaluable possession—the most primal of our senses.

Blending Notes

◉

TOP NOTES: Grapefruit, Hyssop Decumbens, Lemon, Lime, Mandarin, Orange, Peppermint, Ravensara Aromatica, Spearmint, Tangerine

MIDDLE NOTES: Cabreuva, Cassia Bark, Chamomile (Roman), Champaca Flower, Cinnamon Leaf, Clary Sage, Clove Bud, Cypress, Eucalyptus Citriodora, Fennel (Sweet), Geranium, Gingergrass, Guaiacwood, Havozo Bark, Helichrysum, Juniper Berries, Lavender, Litsea Cubeba, Manuka, Marjoram, Myrtle, Neroli, Pimento Berry, Rosemary, Sage, Spruce, Thyme, Ylang-Ylang

BASE NOTES: Ambrette Seed, Amyris, Cedarwood (Atlas), Copaiba, Patchouli, Rose, Sandalwood, Spikenard, Vanilla

Blending Essential Oils

Each essential oil has its own unique properties and benefits. When combined correctly with other essential oils, the synergism of the blend cannot only produce a better aroma, but also make it more efficacious. For instance, a person wants to use peppermint oil for massage in the wintertime. But the menthol in the peppermint causes a cooling effect. Since we want to avoid cooling the body when the weather is cold, we can add gingergrass and sandalwood oil to the peppermint to balance out the temperature and improve the effectiveness of the massage. Another example is when a person enjoys the fragrance of vanilla and wants to use it during the daytime. Vanilla can calm and relax a person to the point of becoming sleepy, so adding spearmint and gingergrass oils to it make a more-balanced blend.

A well-balanced blend is composed of base, middle, and top notes. The top notes are the first to be noticed, since they are the most volatile

CAMPHORACEOUS

Hyssop Decumbens	Marjoram
Myrtle	Ravensara
Rosemary	Aromatica
	Sage

CITRUS

Eucalyptus Citriodora	Grapefruit
Lemon	Lime
Litsea Cubeba	Mandarin
Orange	Tangerine

EARTHY

Patchouli	Spikenard

FLORAL

Champaca Flower	Geranium
Neroli	Rose
Ylang-Ylang	

HERBACEOUS

Chamomile (Roman)	Clary Sage
Gingergrass	Lavender

LICORICE

Fennel (Sweet)	Havozo Bark

MINTY

Peppermint	Spearmint

MUSKY

Ambrette Seed

SPICY

Cinnamon Leaf	Clove Bud
Pimento Berry	Marjoram
Thyme	

SWEET

Cassia Bark	Champaca
Guaiacwood	Flower
Manuka	Helichrysum
Vanilla	Spruce
	Ylang-Ylang

TURPENTINE-LIKE

Cypress	Fir Needles
Juniper Berry	

WOODY

Amyris	Cabreuva
Cedarwood (Atlas)	Copaiba
Sandalwood	

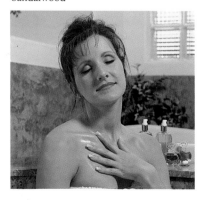

and dissipate the quickest. The middle notes, longer lasting than the top notes, add richness and body. The base notes are the longest lasting. They hold together and give staying power and fullness to the overall aroma.

Aromatic Air Fragrancing

People involved in aromatic fragrancing have no doubt about its effectiveness. In Japan, when fragrant oils are diffused in the workplace, companies report an increase in productivity and a decrease in absenteeism. In one study, typing errors were reduced by 20% when lavender oil was diffused, by 33% with jasmine, and by 54% with lemon oil.

When we walk into a person's home, one of the first things we notice are the odors. They give an impression of the people living there and what is taking place in the house—if they are cooking, baking, smoking, cleaning, or painting. Even the odors of pets can be quite easily detected.

Air freshener mist sprays and diffusers can help fragrance the home environment to remove odors and affect people in a positive way. Just as we experience elevated moods from smelling the beautiful outdoor fragrances of flowers and the fresh forest air, we can re-create these wonderful scents in our home to enhance our lives.

In the kitchen, many odors are produced—some pleasant, others not. The air freshener needs to be strong enough to overcome the lingering odors produced from cooking, baking, or broiling highly odorous foods, such as garlic, onions, fish, and mushrooms. In the dining area, you may want to use an air freshener that is pleasing and helps people to enjoy the meal. The living room should have a lively fragrance to encourage happiness and conversation, while the bedroom needs a calming and relaxing aroma. In the workroom, the best freshener is one providing a cheerful atmosphere and mental clarity. The bathroom fragrance should be fresh and clean with antiseptic properties. Please see Chapter 7 for the Room Air Fragrancing formulas.

Methods of Use

Application

The self-application method is used when there isn't another person available to give a massage, or when a massage is not necessary. The oils should be rubbed into the skin until they are fully absorbed. Then apply and rub a small amount of arrowroot or cornstarch powder onto the area to remove any remaining oil from the skin.

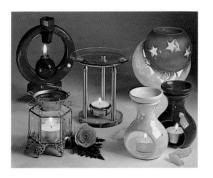

Aroma Lamps

There are a variety of beautiful and decorative aroma lamps to use as a showpiece in the home or at the office.

To use: Fill the small container on top of the aroma lamp with water and add the essential oils. Depending on the type of aroma lamp you have, light the candle or turn on the lightbulb. As the water heats, the fragrance of the oil diffuses into the air.

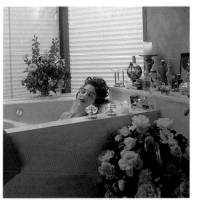

Baths

Soaking in warm water scented with essential oils can be so pleasurable that once you experience an aromatic bath, plain-water baths will become a thing of the past.

To prepare for your bath, select one of the bath oil formulas in Chapter 7. Close the bathroom door and window to keep the warm steam of the bathwater and essential oil vapors from escaping out of the room. Then fill the bathtub with water as warm as you like and turn on soft music. Mix the essential oils with the carrier oil and pour the formula into the bathwater. Swirl the water to distribute the oils evenly throughout the tub and enter the bath immediately. Enjoy the wonderful aromas!

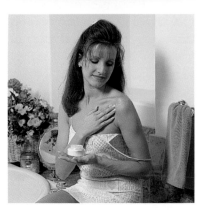

Body Powders

Body powders are used to scent and deodorize the skin.

To prepare: Measure the amount of arrowroot powder or cornstarch needed, then pour into a small wide-mouthed glass jar. Add the essential oils, mix the ingredients thoroughly, and tightly cap the jar. Allow the powder to sit for a day before use. Store in a dark, cool place.

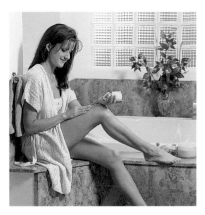

Cremes

Cremes help nourish and moisturize the skin, and assist in bringing about soft and beautiful-looking skin. They apply easily and have a smooth texture. Natural cocoa butter and shea butter are used in the creme formulas in this book.

To prepare: Place the indicated amount of the vegetable butter into a wide-mouthed glass jar, put the jar into a small pot of water, and heat on a low flame. When the butter melts, add the carrier oil, mix well, and remove from the heat. As the mixture cools, add the essential oils, stir well, and tightly cap the jar. Wait until the creme cools completely and becomes creamy in texture before using. Store in a dark, cool place.

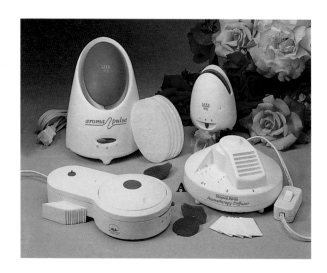

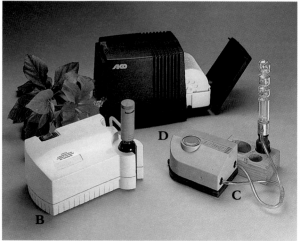

Diffusers

Diffusers disperse a mist of essential-oil microparticles, which creates an aromatic atmosphere for the indoors. There are different types of diffusers on the market. You can choose a smaller or larger unit, depending on the size of the area to be fragranced. The formulas given for diffuser use in Chapter 7 are in percentages rather than drops because of the different types of units. (A): Essential oils are added to a pad and warmed by an electrical heating element that diffuses the aroma into the air. (B & C): Essential oils are placed in a small glass bottle. The oil is then propelled into a nebulizer and vaporized into the air. (D): Cold water is added into a slide-out container, and then essential oils are added to the water. The fan disperses the aroma vapors into the air.

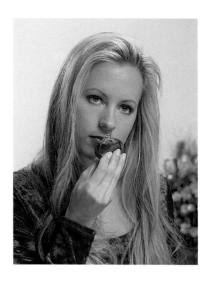

Inhalers

Inhalers are convenient to use and provide quick results.

To prepare: Combine the essential oils in a small ¼ ounce (7.5 ml) or ½ ounce (15 ml) glass bottle with a wide opening. Tighten the cap and gently shake to mix the oils.

To use: Relax in a comfortable chair, open the bottle, and slowly inhale the vapors 15–20 times. Breathe deeply. Cap the bottle immediately after use and store for the next time.

Over a period of time the inhaler may lose its potency as the vapors become faint. At that point, there is no need to discard the oils. Instead, reuse the oils by combining them in a fine-mist spray bottle with purified water and adding fresh essential oils to use as a mist spray.

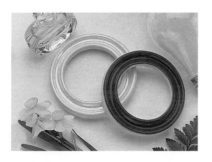

Lightbulb Rings

Place the lightbulb ring on top of a cool lightbulb and carefully drop the essential oil(s) into the circular groove of the ring. Please make sure not to get any oil on the lightbulb. Turn on the light and, as the bulb becomes heated, the aromatic fragrance will be diffused into the air. Use only lightbulbs of 60 watts or less.

Massage

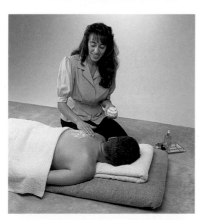

One of the most simple pleasures in life is receiving an aromatherapy massage in a relaxed, peaceful ambience with a comfortable temperature setting and soft music playing in the background. Taking time out to experience this wonderful, nurturing form of touch in a tranquil environment can be beneficial to improve health and overall well-being.

For best results when giving a massage, please follow these guidelines:

- Wear comfortable clothing.
- Fingernails should be short.
- A massage table or a firm cushion can be placed on the floor to do the massage on.
- Be in a calm and positive state of mind, since tension can easily be transferred to the receiver during the massage.
- A spray mist can be used prior to the receiver coming into the room.
- Choose the appropriate massage formula and place all oils nearby to avoid searching for them during the massage.
- Wash hands with warm water before and after giving the massage.
- Warm the carrier oil by placing the small container in warm water. Pour an ample amount into the palm of your hand, rub hands together, and then apply the oil on the receiver's skin.
- After the massage, use arrowroot powder or cornstarch to dry off any remaining oil on the skin.

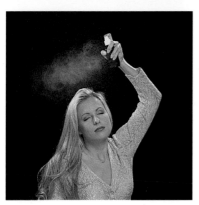

Mist Sprays

A convenient and effective way to disperse aromatic vapors in the air is through the use of a mist spray. As the aromas mature in the bottle, the fragrance improves.

To prepare: Fill a fine-mist spray bottle with purified water, add the essential oils, and tightly cap the bottle.

To use: Shake the bottle well. Sit comfortably in a chair. Position the sprayer so that the mist falls in front of your face. Close your eyes and spray approximately ten times over the head. Stop with every two to three sprays and inhale deeply. Store in a dark, cool place.

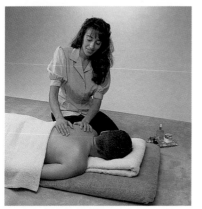

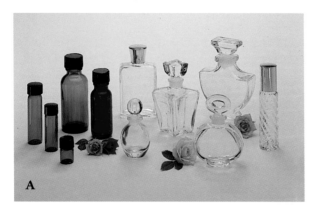

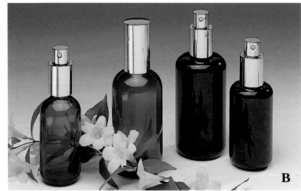

Supplies and Accessories

These are the necessary supplies and accessories used to mix and store the blends in Chapter 7. Dark-colored glass bottles are recommended for use; however, the clear glass bottles can be used for display purposes so that the color of the oils can be seen.

(A) Bottles for essential oils.

(B & C) Bottles with fine-mist sprayers.

(D) Assorted bottles with fine-mist sprayers and dispensing pumps.

(E) Bottles with dispensing pumps.

(F) Jars for cremes and powder blends.

(G) Handy small-sized bottles with fine-mist sprayers and dispensers.

(H) Glass droppers and funnel.

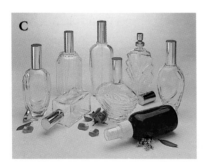

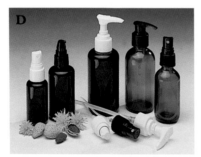

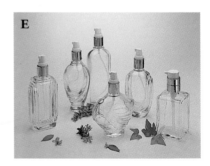

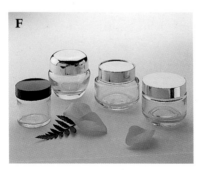

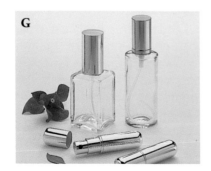

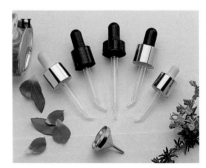

Safe Use and Storage of Oils

Please follow these guidelines for the safe and proper use of the essential oils:

- Dilute essential oils in a carrier oil before applying on the skin. This is necessary to prevent the possibility of skin irritation. Should any irritation occur as a result of the essential oils, apply additional carrier oil. Lavender oil can also be used to quickly soothe the area. If irritation persists, discontinue the use of the formula.
- Take extra care not to get the oils or vapors in the eyes. If this occurs, flush with cool water.
- Many essential oils should not be used during pregnancy due to the stimulating effect they have on the urinary system and uterus. The oils can be helpful just before labor to facilitate the onset of childbirth. However, if used in the early months of pregnancy, they can bring on contractions with the possibility of premature delivery. Small amounts (two to three drops at one time) of the following essential oils contained in this book are safe during pregnancy: Cypress, Geranium, Grapefruit, Lavender, Lemon, Lime, Mandarin, Neroli, Orange, Patchouli, Sandalwood, Spearmint, Tangerine, Ylang-Ylang. Sesame oil can be used as a carrier oil.
- For women nursing their babies, please use extra care in the selection of essential oils, especially for skin application, since the effects of the oils are transferred to the infant.
- If a person is highly allergic, this simple and easy test can be done: Rub a drop of carrier oil on the upper chest area. In 12 hours, check for redness on the skin or any other reaction. If the skin is clear, place one drop of an essential oil in twenty drops of the same carrier oil that was tested to be safe and again rub the mixture on the upper chest area. If there is no skin reaction after 12 hours, both the carrier and essential oil should be fine to use.
- Do not consume alcohol, except for a small glass of wine with a meal, in the time period when using essential oils.
- Do not use the essential oils while on medication, since the oils might interfere with the medicine.
- The following oils contained in this book can be especially irritating to the skin and must be used with extra care, particularly by those with dry skin: Cinnamon Leaf, Clove Bud, Fennel (Sweet), Gingergrass, Grapefruit, Lemon, Lime, Litsea Cubeba, Mandarin, Orange, Peppermint, Pimento Berry, Spearmint, Tangerine, and Thyme. Cassia Bark should not be used on the skin.
- When using citrus, phototoxic, and other essential oils that can irritate the skin, avoid sunbathing or using the sauna/steam room for at least 4 hours.
- There are people with extremely sensitive skin who cannot tolerate

Helpful Measurements

❧

2 tablespoons = 1 ounce = 30 ml

1 tablespoon = ½ ounce = 15 ml

3 teaspoons = ½ ounce = 15 ml

1 teaspoon = 5 ml

28.35 grams = 1 ounce

14.17 grams = 1 tablespoon

4.73 grams = 1 teaspoon

the essential oils without having skin irritation. If this is the case, please discontinue use.

- If spilled on furniture, many essential oils will remove the finish; therefore, be careful when handling the bottles.
- Light and oxygen cause oils to deteriorate rapidly. Refrigeration does not prevent spoilage but diminishes the speed at which it occurs. Therefore, oils should be stored in amber-colored glass bottles in a dark and cool place.
- Always use a glass dropper when measuring drops of essential oil.
- Keep all bottles tightly closed to prevent the oils from evaporating and oxidizing.
- After mixing carrier and essential oils together, use as soon as possible or within a 6-month period to avoid the possibility of spoilage.
- Always store essential oils out of sight and reach of children.
- Clearly label all bottles and jars that contain blends.

Common Mistakes

In order to obtain maximum results, it is important to avoid these commonly made mistakes:

1. Not fully massaging the formulas into the skin. The oils should be massaged in for at least 30 minutes.
2. Wiping off the oil that remains on the skin after a massage or application with a tissue or towel. Instead, rub in cornstarch or arrowroot powder to dry off the remaining oil from the skin.
3. Not inhaling deeply the vapors from the inhaler and mist spray formulas. By not inhaling deeply, hardly any vapors enter the breathing passages.
4. Not misting the mist sprays properly. It is important that the mist falls in front of the face with eyes closed.
5. Using stimulating essential oils before bedtime.
6. Using sleep-inducing essential oils during the daytime.
7. Carelessly applying essential oils near the eyes and other sensitive areas of the body. Irritation can result, causing discomfort.
8. Leaving bottles of oils exposed to direct light and not using dark-colored glass bottles to store oils in. The effectiveness of the oils is reduced when they are improperly stored.

Chapter 4
Experiencing Aromatherapy

Many people become greatly intrigued after smelling the aromas of the essential oils, but there's so much more to be experienced. When used regularly, the oils can affect us on our deepest levels by lifting the spirit, awakening the senses, stirring emotions, touching the heart, and enlivening every part of our being. Some oils work instantly, others are more subtle and take longer; some will warm you on a cold winter day, while others will cool you in the heat of the summer; the energizing oils are best used early in the day, while the relaxants are best before bedtime; some of the aromas are instantly liked, others take time to get used to. In due time with experience, you will be able to select the oils that are right for each occasion.

You may start to notice some very interesting occurrences taking place as you do this exercise. Certain aromas may trigger memories you hadn't thought of in a while: some enjoyable, others perhaps you need to deal with.

Some people may discover that they are so wound up with stress that, as they start to calm down, they may feel uneasy and actually resist becoming relaxed. If this is the case, give yourself permission to release your stress and try one of the *Peace and Calm* or *Soothe Nervous Tension* formulas. The more you practice, the easier it will become.

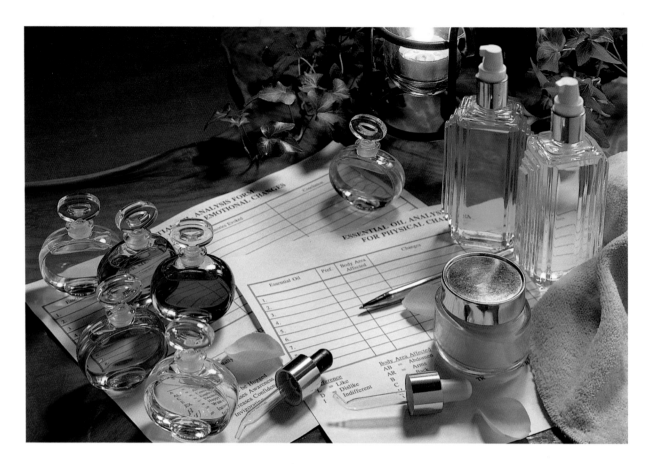

Aromatherapy encourages us to gain greater understanding of how scents affect us. Explore, learn, discover, and involve yourself. Get acquainted with many of the scents you are currently unfamiliar with. Allow your senses to be taken on a fascinating journey and be open to enjoying more of the simple pleasures in life. Observe, pay close attention to your feelings, mood, and passing thoughts, and don't overlook the vital importance of the messages the scents bring.

To understand and fully appreciate how each individual essential oil affects you, set up the following items and do the exercise.

Items Needed

- Carrier oil
- Essential oils
- Glass droppers
- Arrowroot powder or cornstarch
- A pen or pencil
- Make a copy of the *Essential Oil Analysis Form for Mental, Mood & Emotional Changes* and *Essential Oil Analysis for Physical Changes* in this chapter.

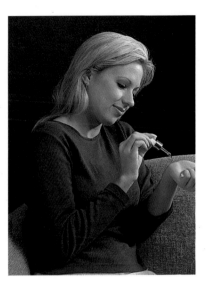
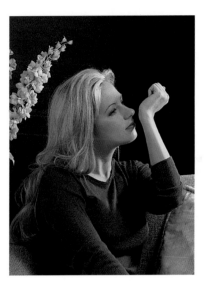

Words to Describe Scents

Balsamic

Bitter

Camphoraceous

Citrusy

Earthy

Floral

Fresh

Fruity

Herbaceous

Irritating

Lemony

Minty

Musky

Musty

Orangy

Penetrating

Piercing

Pungent

Refreshing

Salty

Smokey

Spicy

Sweet

Vaporous

Woody

Instructions

1. Find a peaceful and comfortable room to relax in. Make sure you won't be disturbed by the telephone, doorbell, people, or pets entering the room.
2. Play soft music (optional) to help create a relaxing mood.
3. Place the items necessary for this analysis exercise near where you will be sitting.
4. Add a feeling of tranquillity to the room by adjusting the lighting.
5. Relax in a comfortable chair or on a cushion on the floor.
6. Apply approximately twenty drops of carrier oil on your wrist and forearm. The carrier oil should coat the entire skin area. Gently rub both wrists together to evenly distribute the oil.
7. Select an essential oil and apply one drop over the carrier oil on one of your wrists and gently rub the oil into the skin. Close your eyes and bring your wrist up toward your nose without touching your face or nostrils. Slowly inhale the vapors. Sit quietly for 5–10 minutes. Clear your mind, relax your body, and focus on the benefits of the oil according to the categories listed on the worksheets. The more you relax, the easier it will be for you to experience the effects of the essential oil.
8. Fill out both Essential Oil Analysis forms.
9. To dull the scent on the skin from one oil to another, rub in a small amount of powder over the area where the previous essential oil was applied. To evaluate the next essential oil, repeat instructions #6 and #7.

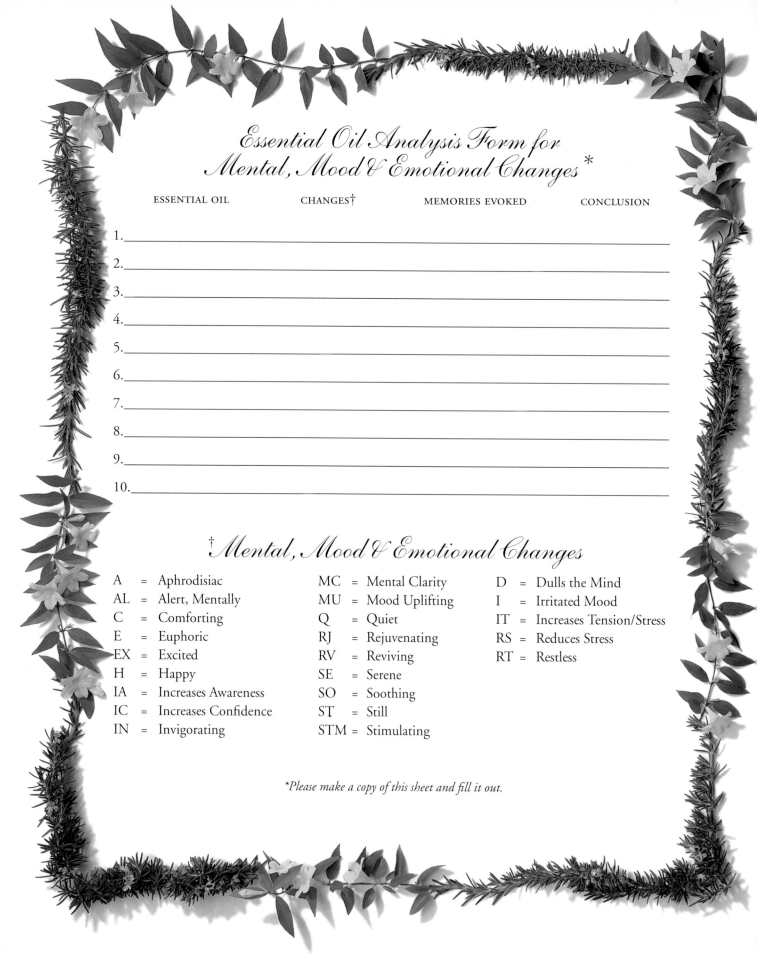

Essential Oil Analysis Form for
Mental, Mood & Emotional Changes *

	ESSENTIAL OIL	CHANGES†	MEMORIES EVOKED	CONCLUSION
1.				
2.				
3.				
4.				
5.				
6.				
7.				
8.				
9.				
10.				

† Mental, Mood & Emotional Changes

A	=	Aphrodisiac	MC	=	Mental Clarity	D	= Dulls the Mind
AL	=	Alert, Mentally	MU	=	Mood Uplifting	I	= Irritated Mood
C	=	Comforting	Q	=	Quiet	IT	= Increases Tension/Stress
E	=	Euphoric	RJ	=	Rejuvenating	RS	= Reduces Stress
EX	=	Excited	RV	=	Reviving	RT	= Restless
H	=	Happy	SE	=	Serene		
IA	=	Increases Awareness	SO	=	Soothing		
IC	=	Increases Confidence	ST	=	Still		
IN	=	Invigorating	STM	=	Stimulating		

Please make a copy of this sheet and fill it out.

Essential Oil Analysis Form for Physical Changes *

ESSENTIAL OIL	PREF.	BODY AREA AFFECTED	CHANGES	BODY TEMP.	WEIGHT SENSATION	COMMENTS
1.						
2.						
3.						
4.						
5.						
6.						
7.						
8.						
9.						
10.						

PREFERENCE
L = Like
D = Dislike
I = Indifferent

BODY AREA AFFECTED
AB = Abdomen
AR = Arms
B = Back
C = Chest
H = Head
L = Legs
N = Neck
S = Spine

CHANGES
BE = Breathing Easier
C = Calming
E = Energizing
IT = Increased Tension
ML = Muscle Loosener
P = Pain Relief
TR = Tension Relief

BODY TEMPERATURE
C = Cooling
W = Warming
NC = No Change

WEIGHT SENSATION
L = Light Body Feeling
H = Heavy Body Feeling
NC = No Change

* Please make a copy of this sheet and fill it out.

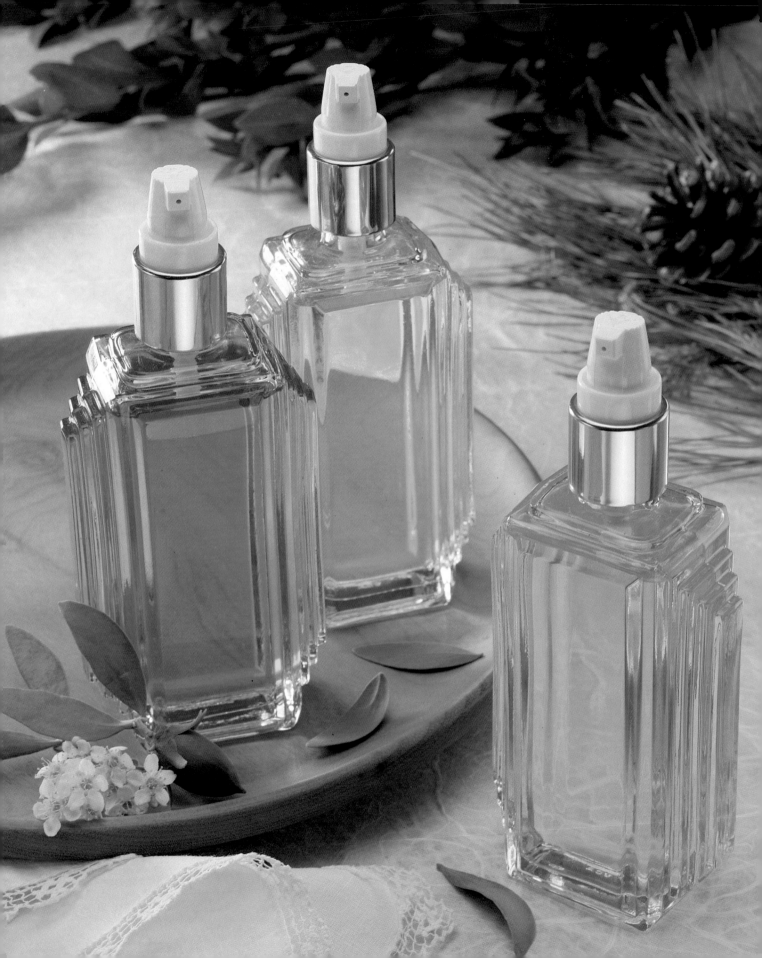

Chapter 5
Carrier Oils

In aromatherapy, carrier oils play a key role by diluting the essential oils for use in massage, skin, and hair care preparations. These oils are beneficial in protecting the skin by moisturizing, soothing, softening, and nourishing the skin cells as the oil gets absorbed deep into the skin layers. Whenever essential oils are applied topically, carrier oils must be combined to form a blend.

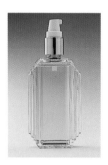

Almond (Sweet)
Botanical Name: *Prunus amygdalus, P. dulcis*
Family: *Rosaceae*
The oil is extracted from the nuts of the tree.
Plant Description: Sweet almond is a tree that grows to a height of about 35 feet (10.6 meters), and has pinkish-white flowers, followed by green fruits, each containing a nut.

AROMATHERAPY USES
Skin and hair care; moisturizing.

Avocado
Botanical Name: *Persea americana, P. gratissima*
Family: *Lauraceae*
The oil is extracted from the kernels and fruits of the tree.

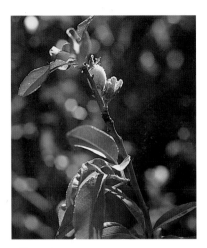

Almond

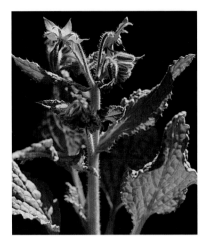

Borage

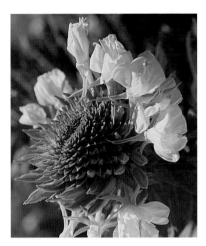

Evening Primrose

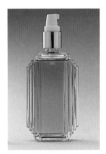

Plant Description: Avocado is an evergreen tree that grows to a height of about 30–60 feet (9–18 meters), and has dark green oval leaves and greenish yellow flowers that develop into yellow, green, red, or purple fruit. The pulp is soft and buttery with a large kernel inside.

AROMATHERAPY USES
Skin and hair care; moisturizing; purifying to the skin.
Comments: For massage blends, it is best to mix approximately 20% of avocado oil with another carrier oil. For skin and hair care purposes, avocado oil can be applied without being diluted.

Borage

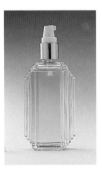

Botanical Name: *Borago officinalis*
Family: *Boraginaceae*
The oil is extracted from the seeds of the plant.
Plant Description: Borage is a plant that grows to a height of about 2–4 feet (0.6–1.2 meters), and has large pointed oval leaves, hairy stems, and star-shaped, blue flowers with a dark stamen in the center. The scent of the plant is similar to a cucumber.

AROMATHERAPY USES
Calming; helps reduce premenstrual stress; relieves menstrual pain; reduces inflammation.
Skin and hair care; moisturizing; soothes inflamed skin.
Comments: For massage blends, it is best to mix approximately 20% of borage oil with another carrier oil. For skin and hair care purposes, borage oil can be applied without being diluted.

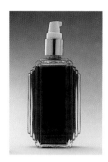

Calophyllum (Tamanu)
Botanical Name: *Calophyllum inophyllum*
Family: *Guttiferae*
The oil is extracted from the kernels of the fruits of the tree.
Plant Description: Calophyllum is an evergreen tree that grows to a height of about 100 feet (30 meters), and has sweet, fragrant white flowers that develop into fruits, which have a thin pulp and a taste similar to an apple.

AROMATHERAPY USES
Skin and hair care; soothing to the skin.
Comments: For massage oil blends, it is best to mix approximately 50% of calophyllum oil with another carrier oil. For skin and hair care purposes, calophyllum oil can be applied without being diluted.

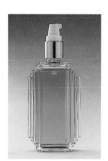

Carrot Root (Heliocarrot)
Botanical Name: *Daucus carota*
Family: *Apiaceae*
The oil is extracted from the roots of the plant.
Plant Description: Carrot is a plant that grows to a height of about 1 foot (0.3 meters), and has feathery leaves and white flower heads.

AROMATHERAPY USES
Skin and hair care; moisturizing; rejuvenates brittle, dry hair.
Comments: For massage oil blends, it is best to mix approximately 20% of carrot oil with another carrier oil. For skin and hair care purposes, carrot oil can be applied without being diluted.

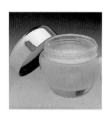

Cocoa Butter
Botanical Name: *Theobroma cacao*
Family: *Sterculiaceae*
The butter is extracted from the beans of the tree.
Plant Description: Cocoa is an evergreen tree that grows to a height of about 24 feet (7.3 meters), and has large glossy leaves and small yellow flowers that develop into yellow or red fruits, containing many beanlike seeds.

AROMATHERAPY USES
Stimulant to the body.
Skin and hair care; moisturizing.

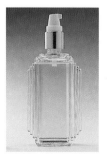

Evening Primrose
Botanical Name: *Oenothera biennis*
Family: *Onagraceae*
The oil is extracted from the seeds of the plant.
Plant Description: Evening primrose is a plant that grows to a height of about 1–8 feet (0.3–2.4 meters), and has long pointed leaves and many fragrant yellow flowers that open at dusk to attract night-flying insects

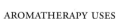

for pollination. Following the flowers are capsules containing many small brownish-colored seeds.

AROMATHERAPY USES
Helps reduce premenstrual stress; relieves menstrual pain; reduces inflammation.
Skin and hair care; moisturizing; soothing to the skin.
Comments: For massage blends, it is best to mix approximately 20% evening primrose with another carrier oil. For skin and hair purposes, evening primrose oil can be applied without being diluted.

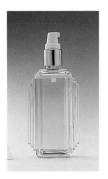

Grapeseed
Botanical Name: *Vitis vinifera*
Family: *Vitaceae*
The oil is extracted from the seeds of the fruit of the plant.
Plant Description: The grape plant is a climbing vine that grows to about 30 feet (9 meters), and has small green flowers that develop into bunches of sweet-flavored green or purple fruits.

AROMATHERAPY USES
Skin and hair care.

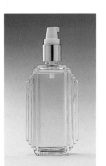

Jojoba
Botanical Name: *Simmondsia chinensis*
Family: *Buxaceae*
The vegetable wax/oil is extracted from the seeds of the shrub.
Plant Description: Jojoba is an evergreen shrub that grows to a height of about 3–18 feet (0.9–5.5 meters), and has small leathery leaves. The male flowers are yellow; the female flowers are green and develop into olive-shaped fruits containing seeds inside. The male and female flowers grow on separate plants.

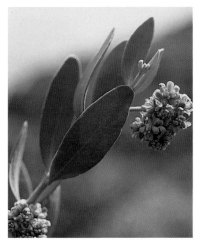

Jojoba (bloom)

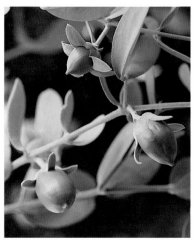

Jojoba (fruit)

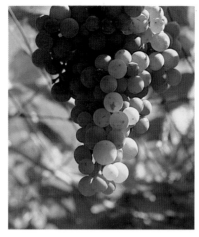
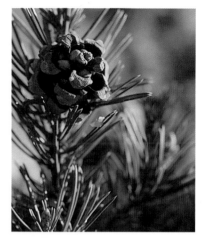

Grapeseed   *Pine Nut*

AROMATHERAPY USES

Skin and hair care; moisturizing; helps to reduce stretch marks; suntanning oil for those who tend to burn easily in the sun.

Comments: For massage blends, it is best to mix approximately 50% jojoba oil with another carrier oil. For skin and hair care purposes, jojoba oil can be applied without being diluted.

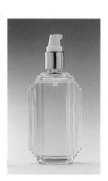

Kukui Nut

Botanical Name: *Aleurites moluccana*
Family: *Euphorbiaceae*
The oil is extracted from the nuts of the tree.
Plant Description: Kukui nut is an evergreen tree that grows to a height of about 70 feet (21 meters), and has small white flowers that develop into fruits containing the nut inside.

AROMATHERAPY USES

Skin and hair care; balances, rejuvenates, and softens the skin.

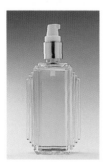

Macadamia Nut

Botanical Name: *Macadamia integrifolia*
Family: *Protoceae*
The oil is extracted from the nuts of the tree.
Plant Description: Macadamia is an evergreen tree that grows to a height of about 30–70 feet (9–21 meters), and has shiny leaves. Its white flowers develop into nuts.

AROMATHERAPY USES

Skin and hair care; softens and restores the skin.

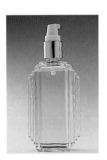

Pine Nut

Botanical Name: *Pinus edulis, P. pinea*
Family: *Pinaceae*
The oil is extracted from the nuts of the tree.
Plant Description: The *Pinus edulis* tree grows to a height of about 50 feet (15 meters), and has dark green needlelike leaves and greenish-brown cones with nuts inside. The *Pinus pinea* tree grows to a height of about 80 feet (24 meters), and has green needlelike leaves and brown cones with nuts inside.

AROMATHERAPY USES
Skin and hair care; soothing and healing to the skin tissues.

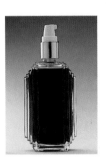

Pistachio Nut

Botanical Name: *Pistacia vera*
Family: *Anacardiaceae*
The oil is extracted from the nuts of the tree.
Plant Description: Pistachio is a tree that grows to a height of about 30–40 feet (9–12 meters). The male and female flowers are produced on different trees.

AROMATHERAPY USES
Skin and hair care; moisturizing.

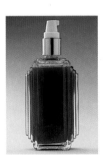

Sea Buckthorn Berry

Botanical Name: *Hippophae rhamnoides*
Family: *Elaeagnaceae*
The oil is extracted from the berries of the shrub.
Plant Description: Sea buckthorn is a shrub that grows to a height of about 30 feet (9 meters), and has clusters of small yellow flowers that develop into small orange berries.

AROMATHERAPY USES
Warming; improves circulation; relaxing; promotes a restful sleep; mood uplifting; loosens tight muscles.
Skin, hair, and nail care; soothing and healing to the skin; moisturizes chapped lips.
Comments: For massage blends, it is best to mix approximately 50% sea buckthorn oil with another carrier oil. For skin, hair, and nail care purposes, sea buckthorn oil can be applied without being diluted.

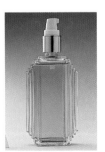

Sesame

Botanical Name: *Sesamum indicum*
Family: *Pedaliaceae*
The oil is extracted from the seeds of the plant.
Plant Description: Sesame is a plant that grows to a height of about 3–6 feet (0.9–2 meters), and has oval leaves and white or pink tubular flowers

with purple spots that develop into white, yellow, red, brown, or black seeds.

AROMATHERAPY USES
Skin and hair care; moisturizing; soothing to the skin.

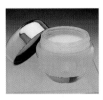

Shea Butter
Botanical Name: *Butyrosperum parkii*
Family: *Sapotaceae*
The butter is extracted from the kernels of the tree.
Plant Description: Shea is a tree that grows to a height of about 70 feet (21 meters), and has sweet, fragrant white flowers that develop into brown fruit with a large white kernel inside.

AROMATHERAPY USES
Skin and hair care; moisturizing; used as a suntan creme.

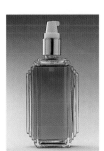

Sisymbrium
Botanical Name: *Sisymbrium officinale*
Family: *Brassicaceae*
The oil is extracted from the seeds of the plant.
Plant Description: Sisymbrium, also known as hedge mustard, is a plant that grows to a height of about 4 feet (1 meter), and has small yellow flowers, followed by pods containing seeds that resemble mustard seeds.

AROMATHERAPY USES
Skin and hair care; moisturizing; softens the skin; improves the complexion; reduces wrinkles.
Comments: For massage blends, it is best to mix approximately 50% of sisymbrium oil with another carrier oil. For skin and hair care purposes, sisymbrium oil can be applied without being diluted.

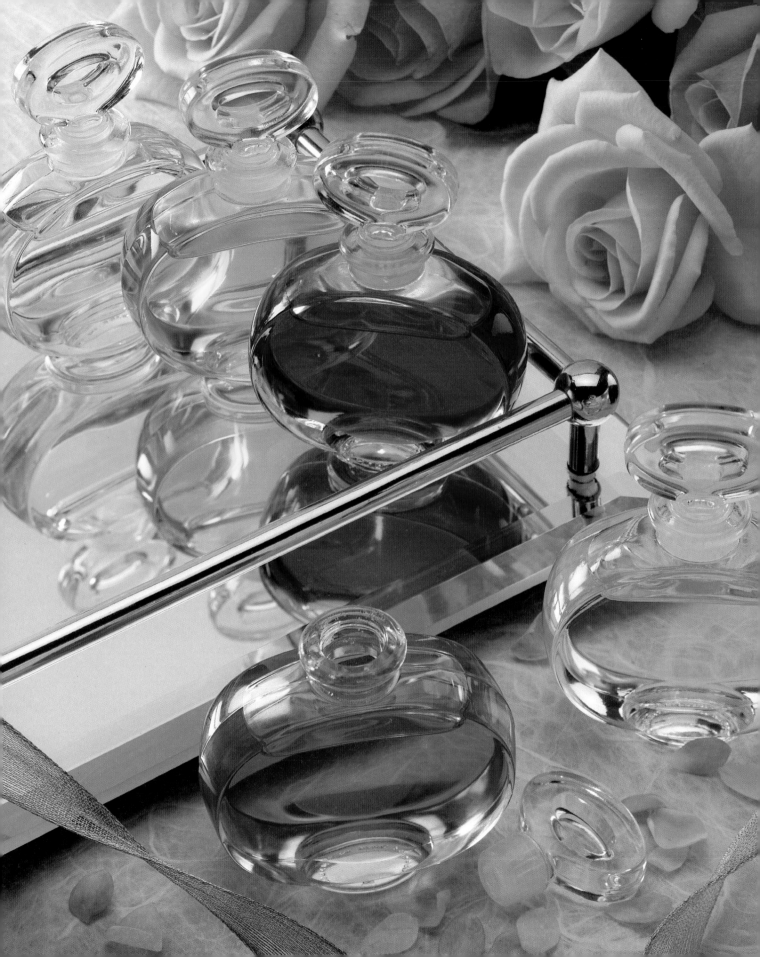

Chapter 6
Essential Oils

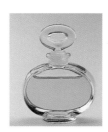

Ambrette Seed

Botanical Name: *Abelmoschus moschatus, Hibiscus abelmoschus*
Family: *Malvaceae*
The essential oil is extracted from the seeds of the shrub.
Scent of the oil: Musky, sweet
Plant Description: Hibiscus is an evergreen shrub that grows to a height of about 5 feet (1.5 meters), and has large yellow flowers with purple centers, or large red flowers with white centers. The fruit is an oblong seedpod that splits at the tip when it matures. The seeds are gray-brown with a musklike scent and the oil produced from them is called ambrette seed oil.

AROMATHERAPY USES
Calming, reduces stress and nervous tension; mood uplifting; lessens aches and pains; heals and moisturizes the skin.
Comments: In the formulas given in this book, it is recommended that ambrette seed CO_2 extracted oil be used.
PRECAUTION: Ambrette seed is phototoxic. Avoid exposure to direct sunlight for several hours after applying the oil on the skin.

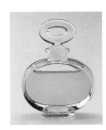

Amyris

Botanical Name: *Amyris balsamifera*
Family: *Rutaceae*
The essential oil is extracted from the wood chips of the tree.
Scent of the oil: Sweet, woody, smokey
Plant Description: Amyris is an evergreen tree that grows to a height of about 60 feet (18 meters), and has clusters of white flowers that develop into an edible bluish-black fruit.

AROMATHERAPY USES
Cooling; calming, reduces anxiety, stress, and tension; promotes a peaceful state; deepens the breathing; reviving; improves mental clarity; loosens tight muscles; used as a fixative to hold the scent of a fragrance.

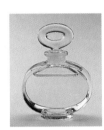

Cabreuva

Botanical Name: *Myrocarpus fastigiatus*
Family: *Fabaceae*
The essential oil is extracted from the wood chips of the tree.
Scent of the oil: Sweet, woody
Plant Description: Cabreuva is a tropical tree that grows to a height of about 50 feet (15 meters).

AROMATHERAPY USES
Warming; calming, reduces stress and tension; helps to breathe easier; mood uplifting, euphoric, aphrodisiac, reviving; improves mental clarity and alertness; loosens tight muscles, reduces pain.

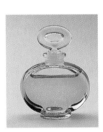

Cassia Bark

Botanical Name: *Cinnamomum aromaticum, C. cassia*
Family: *Lauraceae*
The essential oil is extracted from the bark of the tree.
Scent of the oil: Warm, sweet, rich cinnamon
Plant Description: Cassia is an evergreen tree that grows to a height of about 40–80 feet (12–24 meters), and has a thin-peeling bark, long glossy leathery leaves, and small green flowers that develop into berries, each containing a seed.

AROMATHERAPY USES
Heating, improves circulation; mood uplifting, reviving; lessens pain, increases mobility of the joints; disinfectant; repels insects.
PRECAUTION: Cassia bark oil is heating and can cause skin irritation. It is advisable to avoid use on the skin.

Cedarwood (Atlas)

Botanical Name: *Cedrus atlantica*
Family: *Pinaceae*

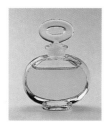

The essential oil is extracted from the wood of the tree.
Scent of the oil: Sweet-floral, woody
Plant Description: Cedarwood is an evergreen tree that grows to a height of about 130–140 feet (39–42.5 meters), and has gray-green needlelike leaves and light green cones that mature to a brownish-gray color.

AROMATHERAPY USES
Cooling; calming, relieves anxiety and nervous tension; promotes a restful sleep, encourages dreaming; helps to breathe easier, opens the sinus and breathing passages, eases chest congestion when rubbed on the chest; improves mental clarity; helpful for meditation; loosens tight muscles, lessens pain; repels insects.

Chamomile (Roman)

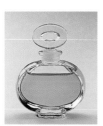

Botanical Name: *Anthemis nobilis, Chamaemelum nobile*
Family: *Asteraceae*
The essential oil is extracted from the flowers and leaves of the plant.
Scent of the oil: Sweet applelike, herbaceous
Plant Description: Roman chamomile grows to a height of about 1 foot (0.3 meters), and has feathery leaves and white flowers with a yellow disk in the center, similar in appearance to daisies.

AROMATHERAPY USES
Calming; promotes a restful sleep; mood uplifting; improves digestion, soothes the intestines; lessens pain, relieves menstrual discomfort, soothes inflammation; healing to the skin; soothes insect bites.

Champaca Flower

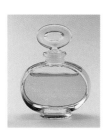

Botanical Name: *Michelia alba, M. champaca*
Family: *Magnoliaceae*
The essential oil is extracted from the flowers of the tree.
Scent of the oil: Sweet-floral
Plant Description: Champaca is an evergreen tree that grows to a height of about 65 feet (19.7 meters), and has long glossy leaves and small fragrant white flowers that develop into fruits containing seeds inside.

AROMATHERAPY USES
Warming; calming, promotes a peaceful state, reduces stress; helps to breathe easier; mood uplifting, euphoric.

Cinnamon Leaf

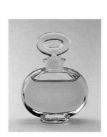

Botanical Name: *Cinnamomum verum, C. zeylanicum*
Family: *Lauraceae*
The essential oil is extracted from the leaves of the tree.
Scent of the oil: Warm, sweet, cinnamon
Plant Description: Cinnamon is a tropical evergreen tree that grows to a height of about 25–60 feet (7.6–18 meters), and has shiny green leath-

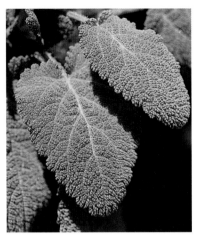

Clary Sage

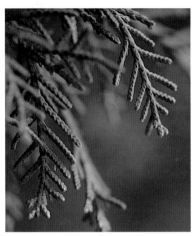

Cypress

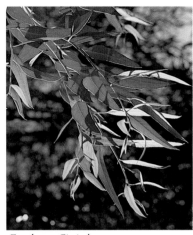

Eucalyptus Citriodora

ery leaves and clusters of small yellow flowers that develop into light blue berries.

AROMATHERAPY USES
Heating, improves circulation; calming, relaxing, reduces stress; mood uplifting, reviving, helps to relieve a fatigued state; improves digestion; purifying, helps to reduce cellulite; loosens tight muscles, lessens pain; disinfectant; repels insects.
PRECAUTION: Cinnamon leaf oil can irritate the skin and should either be avoided or used with extra care by people who have sensitive skin.

Clary Sage

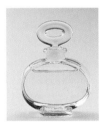

Botanical Name: *Salvia sclarea*
Family: *Lamiaceae*
The essential oil is extracted from the flowering tops of the plant.
Scent of the oil: Sweet, herbaceous
Plant Description: Clary sage is a plant that grows to a height of about 3 feet (0.9 meters), and has whorls of pink, white, or blue flowers, depending on the variety.

AROMATHERAPY USES
Calming, relieves stress and tension; promotes a restful sleep; mood uplifting, aphrodisiac, increases sexual strength; improves digestion; relieves menstrual pain and cramps, regulates the female reproductive system.
PRECAUTION: Due to the relaxing effect of the oil, clary sage should not be used before driving or doing anything that requires full attention. In large amounts, clary sage can be stupefying on the mind. Use small amounts.

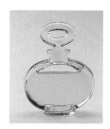

Clove Bud
Botanical Name: *Eugenia aromatica, E. caryophyllata, E. caryophyllus, Syzygium aromaticum*
Family: *Myrtaceae*
The essential oil is extracted from the buds of the tree.
Scent of the oil: Hot-spicy, sweet, penetrating
Plant Description: Clove is a tropical evergreen tree that grows to a height of about 40–70 feet (12–21 meters), and has aromatic dark green leathery leaves and bright pink buds that bloom into yellow flowers, followed by purple berries.

AROMATHERAPY USES
Heating; vapors open sinus and breathing passages; mood uplifting, aphrodisiac, reviving; mental stimulant, improves mental clarity and memory; improves digestion; reduces pain by numbing the area; disinfectant; repels insects.
PRECAUTION: Clove bud oil can irritate the skin and should either be avoided or used with extra care by people who have sensitive skin. Use small amounts.

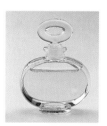

Copaiba
Botanical Name: *Copaifera officinalis*
Family: *Fabaceae*
The essential oil is extracted from the resin of the tree.
Scent of the oil: Sweet, woody
Plant Description: Copaiba is a tropical evergreen tree that grows to a height of about 60 feet (18 meters), and has small yellow flowers followed by fruits that turn from brown to red.

AROMATHERAPY USES
Warming, improves circulation; calming, reduces stress, promotes a peaceful state of mind and a restful sleep; opens the breathing passages, allows deeper breathing; mood uplifting; improves mental clarity and alertness; helpful for meditation; soothes the intestines; healing and moisturizing to the skin; used as a fixative to hold the scent of a fragrance.

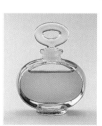

Cypress
Botanical Name: *Cupressus sempervirens*
Family: *Cupressaceae*
The essential oil is extracted from the leaves and twigs of the tree.
Scent of the oil: Turpentine-like, woody, penetrating
Plant Description: Cypress is an evergreen tree that grows to a height of about 80–160 feet (24–48.5 meters), and has dark green leaves, and male and female cones that turn brown when mature.

Balancing to the nervous system; calming, relieves nervous tension and stress; promotes a restful sleep; mood uplifting, refreshing; improves mental clarity and alertness; helpful for the breathing; purifying, helps to reduce cellulite; contracts weak connective tissue; relieves muscle tension; regulates the female reproductive and hormonal systems; lessens perspiration.

Eucalyptus Citriodora

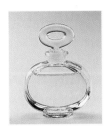

Botanical Name: *Eucalyptus citriodora*
Family: *Myrtaceae*
The essential oil is extracted from the leaves and twigs of the tree.
Scent of the oil: Lemony
Plant Description: Eucalyptus citriodora is an evergreen tree that grows to a height of about 80–170 feet (24–51.5 meters), and has a smooth white bark, narrow pointed leaves with a lemony scent, and white flowers.

AROMATHERAPY USES
Calming; mood uplifting, reviving, helps to relieve a fatigued state.

Fennel (Sweet)

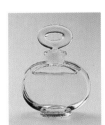

Botanical Name: *Anethum foeniculum, Foeniculum officinale, F. vulgare*
Family: *Apiaceae*
The essential oil is extracted from the seeds of the plant.
Scent of the oil: Warm, fresh, sweet, licorice-like
Plant Description: Fennel is an aromatic plant that grows to a height of about 3–7 feet (0.9–2 meters), and has dark green feathery leaves and clusters of small yellow flowers that develop into brownish-gray seeds.

AROMATHERAPY USES
Warming, improves circulation; reduces stress; promotes a restful sleep; helpful for breathing; improves the digestion, soothes and purifies the intestines, relieves flatulence and aerophagy; purifying, helps to reduce cellulite; relieves pain and menstrual discomfort; increases lactation; disinfectant; repels insects.
PRECAUTION: Due to the toxicity of the oil, use small amounts. Fennel oil can irritate the skin and should either be avoided or used with extra care by people who have sensitive skin. Fennel should not be used by people prone to epileptic seizures or kidney problems.

Fir Needles

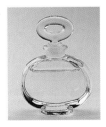

Botanical Name: *Abies alba* (Silver fir), *Abies grandis* (Grand fir), *Abies balsamea* (Fir balsam needles), *Pseudotsuga menziesii* (Douglas fir)
Family: *Pinaceae*
The essential oil is extracted from the needles of the tree.

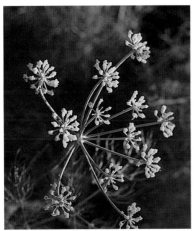

Fennel

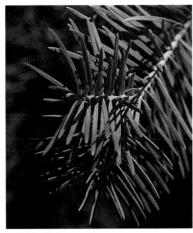

Fir Needles

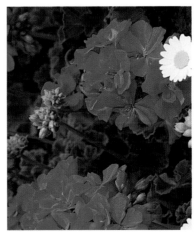

Geranium

Scent of the oil: Fresh, turpentine-like, sweet, balsamic

Plant Description: Fir is an evergreen tree that grows to a height of about 100–300 feet (30–91 meters), and has needlelike leaves, brown cones, and soft and odorless wood. The fir balsam tree is an evergreen that grows to a height of about 40–80 feet (12–24 meters), and has needlelike leaves and purple cones that turn brown when mature.

AROMATHERAPY USES

Calming; the vapors open sinus and breathing passages; mood uplifting, refreshing, reviving; improves mental clarity; encourages communication; purifying, removes lymphatic deposits from the body, helps to reduce cellulite; lessens pain.

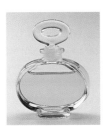

Geranium

Botanical Name: *Pelargonium graveolens*

Family: *Geraniaceae*

The essential oil is extracted from the leaves, stems, and flowers of the plant.

Scent of the oil: Sweet, floral, musty

Plant Description: Geranium is a small fragrant plant that grows to a height of about 3 feet (0.9 meters), and has pink flowers.

AROMATHERAPY USES

Cooling; calming to the nervous system in small amounts, stimulating in large amounts; reduces tension; mood uplifting; encourages communication; stimulates the adrenal glands; purifying, helps to reduce cellulite; lessens pain and inflammation; disinfectant; repels insects; soothes insect bites; kills lice and ticks.

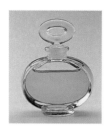

Gingergrass

Botanical Name: *Cymbopogon martinii var. sofia*
Family: *Poaceae*
The essential oil is extracted from the plant, which is a grass.
Scent of the oil: Sharp, vaporous, warm, herbaceous, sweet
Plant Description: Gingergrass is a grass.

AROMATHERAPY USES

Warming, improves circulation; calming, reduces stress; the vapors open sinus and breathing passages; mood uplifting, aphrodisiac, euphoric; improves mental clarity.
PRECAUTION: Gingergrass oil can irritate the skin and should either be avoided or used with extra care by people who have sensitive skin. Use small amounts.

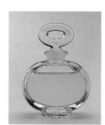

Grapefruit

Botanical Name: *Citrus paradisi*
Family: *Rutaceae*
The essential oil is extracted from the peel of the fruit of the tree.
Scent of the oil: Light, fresh, citrus
Plant Description: Grapefruit is an evergreen citrus tree that grows to a height of about 30–50 feet (9–15 meters), and has glossy green leaves and fragrant white flowers that develop into large edible yellow fruits.

AROMATHERAPY USES

Cooling; reduces stress; mood uplifting, refreshing, reviving; improves mental clarity and awareness, sharpens the senses; increases physical strength and energy; purifying, helps to reduce cellulite and obesity; balances the fluids in the body.
PRECAUTION: Grapefruit oil can irritate the skin and should either be avoided or used with extra care by people who have sensitive skin. Use small amounts. Grapefruit is phototoxic. Avoid exposure to direct sunlight for several hours after applying the oil on the skin.

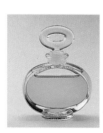

Guaiacwood

Botanical Name: *Bulnesia sarmienti, Guaiacum officinale*
Family: *Zygophyllaceae*
The resin/essential oil is extracted from the wood of the tree.
Scent of the oil: Rich, sweet, fruity, woody
Plant Description: Guaiacwood is an evergreen tree that grows to a height of about 25–40 feet (7.6–12 meters), and has leathery leaves and clusters of blue or purple flowers that develop into seed capsules.

AROMATHERAPY USES

Calming and relaxing, reduces stress and tension; promotes a restful sleep; mood uplifting; improves mental clarity; helpful for meditation;

purifying to the tissues; reduces inflammation, soothes swollen and injured skin tissue; loosens tight muscles.

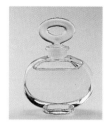

Havozo Bark
Botanical Name: *Cinnamomum camphora, Ravensara anisata*
Family: *Lauraceae*
The essential oil is extracted from the bark of the tree.
Scent of the oil: Fresh licorice-like, warm, sweet, vaporous
Plant Description: Havozo is a small tree.

AROMATHERAPY USES
Warming; calming, reduces stress; promotes a restful sleep; the vapors open the sinus and breathing passages; mood uplifting, euphoric, aphrodisiac; improves mental clarity; encourages communication; soothes the intestines; loosens tight muscles; relieves aches, pains, and menstrual discomfort.

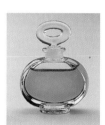

Helichrysum (Everlasting or Immortelle)
Botanical Name: *Helichrysum angustifolium, H. italicum*
Family: *Asteraceae*
The essential oil is extracted from the flowers of the plant.
Scent of the oil: Richly sweet, winelike
Plant Description: Helichrysum is an evergreen plant that grows to a height of about 2 feet (0.6 meters), and has silvery-green leaves and clusters of yellow flowers.

AROMATHERAPY USES
Cooling; relaxing, reduces stress; the vapors open sinus and breathing passages; mood uplifting, euphoric, reviving, strengthening; improves mental clarity and alertness; increases muscle endurance; relieves aches, pains, and menstrual discomfort; disinfectant.

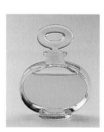

Hyssop Decumbens
Botanical Name: *Hyssopus officinalis var. decumbens*
Family: *Lamiaceae*
The essential oil is extracted from the leaves and flowering tops of the plant.
Scent of the oil: Sweet, camphorous, penetrating vapors
Plant Description: Hyssop is a semi-evergreen bushy plant that grows to a height of about 1–4 feet (0.3–1 meter), and has aromatic leaves and spikes of white, pink, blue, or dark purple flowers.

AROMATHERAPY USES
Relaxing; the vapors open sinus and breathing passages; mood uplifting, reviving; improves mental clarity and alertness.
PRECAUTION: Hyssop decumbens is less toxic and safer to use than the other varieties of hyssop. The oil should not be used by people who are prone epileptic seizures.

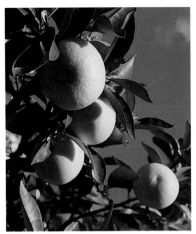
Grapefruit

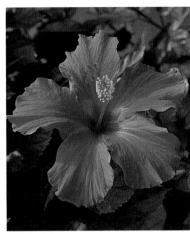
Hibiscus (Ambrette Seed)

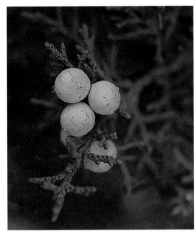
Juniper Berry

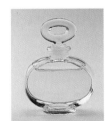

Juniper Berry
Botanical Name: *Juniperus communis*
Family: *Cupressaceae*
The essential oil is extracted from the ripe berries of the bush.
Scent of the oil: Fresh, clean, balsamic, turpentine-like, vaporous
Plant Description: Juniper is an evergreen bush that grows to a height of about 2–6 feet (0.6–2 meters), sometimes reaching as high as 25 feet (7.6 meters). The male trees have yellow cones and the female trees have bluish-green cones. The bluish-green leaves are needlelike. The green berries take 3 years to ripen to a bluish-black color.

AROMATHERAPY USES
Relaxing, reduces stress; mood uplifting, refreshing, reviving; improves mental clarity and memory; purifying, cleansing to the intestines and the tissues in the body, reduces fluid retention, helps to reduce cellulite; lessens pain, painful swellings, painful menstruation; disinfectant; repels insects; soothes insect bites.
PRECAUTION: Due to juniper's strong stimulating effect on the kidneys, use small amounts. Avoid use on a person who has weak kidneys.

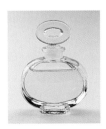

Lavender
Botanical Name: *Lavandula angustifolia, L. officinalis, L. vera*
Family: *Lamiaceae*
The essential oil is extracted from the flowers of the plant.
Scent of the oil: Fresh, herbaceous
Plant Description: Lavender is an aromatic evergreen plant that grows to a height of about 3 feet (0.9 meters), and has spikes of lilac-colored flowers.

AROMATHERAPY USES
Calming; lessens tension; promotes a restful sleep; the vapors open sinus

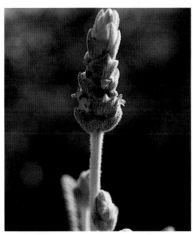

Lavender

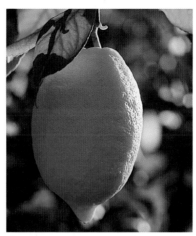

Lemon

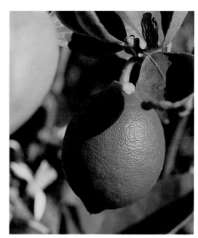

Lime

and breathing passages; mood uplifting; strengthening to the nerves, balances mood swings; improves digestion, soothing to the intestines; purifying, helps to reduce cellulite, gently removes fluid retention; lessens aches and pains, relaxes the muscles, healing to the skin (bruises, cuts, wounds, burns, sunburns, scars, sores, insect bites, and injuries); disinfectant; repels insects, kills lice.

Lemon

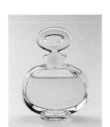

Botanical Name: *Citrus limon*
Family: *Rutaceae*
The essential oil is extracted from the peel of the fruit of the tree.
Scent of the oil: Clean, fresh, lemon-citrus
Plant Description: Lemon is an evergreen citrus tree that grows to a height of about 10–20 feet (3–6 meters), and has fragrant white flowers that develop into edible yellow fruits.

AROMATHERAPY USES
Cooling; calming, relaxing, reduces stress; promotes a restful sleep; mood uplifting, refreshing, reviving; improves mental clarity, alertness, and memory; sharpens the senses; purifying, cleanses the tissues, reduces cellulite and obesity; disinfectant; soothes insect bites.
PRECAUTION: Lemon oil can irritate the skin and should either be avoided or used with extra care by people with sensitive skin. Use small amounts. Lemon is phototoxic. Avoid exposure to direct sunlight for several hours after applying the oil on the skin.

Lime

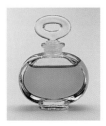

Botanical Name: *Citrus aurantiifolia, C. limetta*
Family: *Rutaceae*
The essential oil is extracted from the peel of the fruit of the tree.
Scent of the oil: Rich, fresh, sweet citrus

Plant Description: Lime is an evergreen citrus tree that grows to a height of about 10–15 feet (3–4.6 meters), and has fragrant small white flowers that develop into edible green fruits.

AROMATHERAPY USES

Cooling; strengthening to the nerves; helpful when there is weakness in the body; reduces stress; mood uplifting, refreshing, reviving; improves mental clarity and alertness, sharpens the senses; purifying, helps to reduce cellulite; disinfectant; soothes insect bites.

PRECAUTION: Lime oil can irritate the skin and should either be avoided or used with extra care by people who have sensitive skin. Use small amounts. Lime is phototoxic. Avoid exposure to direct sunlight for several hours after applying the oil on the skin.

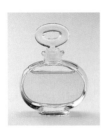

Litsea Cubeba

Botanical Name: *Litsea citrata, L. cubeba*
Family: *Lauraceae*
The essential oil is extracted from the berries of the tree.
Scent of the oil: Rich, heavy, lemonlike
Plant Description: Litsea cubeba is a tropical evergreen tree that grows to a height of about 30 feet (9 meters), and has lemony scented leaves and white flowers that develop into small red or black berries.

AROMATHERAPY USES

Cooling; calming, reduces stress; promotes a restful sleep; mood uplifting, reviving, euphoric; improves mental clarity and alertness; improves digestion; relieves pain.

PRECAUTION: Litsea cubeba oil can irritate the skin and should either be avoided or used with extra care by people who have sensitive skin. Use small amounts.

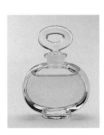

Mandarin

Botanical Name: *Citrus nobilis, C. reticulata*
Family: *Rutaceae*
The essential oil is extracted from the peel of the fruit of the tree.
Scent of the oil: Fresh, sweet-citrus, floral
Plant Description: Mandarin is an evergreen citrus tree that grows to a height of about 20–25 feet (6–7.6 meters), and has glossy leaves and fragrant white flowers that develop into edible orange fruits.

AROMATHERAPY USES

Cooling; calming; promotes a restful sleep; mood uplifting, relieves emotional tension and stress, calms angry and irritable children; improves mental clarity and alertness, sharpens the mind; purifying, helps to reduce cellulite.

PRECAUTION: Mandarin oil can irritate the skin and should either be avoided or used with extra care by people who have sensitive skin. Use small amounts. Mandarin is phototoxic. Avoid exposure to direct sunlight for several hours after applying the oil on the skin.

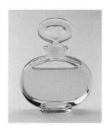

Manuka

Botanical Name: *Leptospermum scoparium*
Family: *Myrtaceae*
The essential oil is extracted from the leaves and branches of the shrub.
Scent of the oil: Richly sweet
Plant Description: Manuka is an evergreen shrub that grows to a height of about 10 feet (3 meters), and has pink, red, or white flowers with a red center.

AROMATHERAPY USES
Calming, reduces stress and tension; helps to breathe easier; mood uplifting, euphoric, aphrodisiac; improves mental clarity; loosens tight muscles; relieves aches and pains; deodorant; disinfectant; healing to the skin.

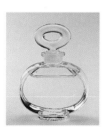

Marjoram (Spanish or Sweet)

Botanical Name: *Thymus mastichina* (Spanish marjoram); *Majorana hortensis, Origanum majorana* (Sweet marjoram)
Family: *Lamiaceae*
The essential oil is extracted from the flowering tops and leaves of the plant.
Scent of the oil: Warm, camphorous, vaporous, spicy
Plant Description: Spanish marjoram is a bushy plant that grows to a height of about 1 foot (0.3 meter), and has small white flowers. Sweet marjoram is a bushy plant that grows to a height of about 2 feet (0.6 meter), and has light grayish-green leaves and white or purple flowers.

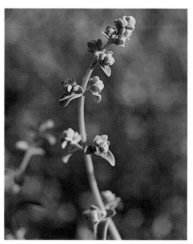

Marjoram

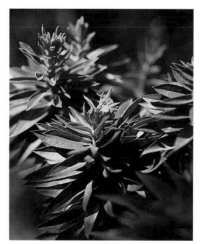

Myrtle

Warming; improves circulation; relaxing, calms nervous tension; promotes a restful sleep; the vapors open sinus and breathing passages, especially helpful during colds and nasal congestion; improves digestion; relaxes tense muscles, relieves aches, pains, painful menstruation, inflammation, and spasms; disinfectant.

PRECAUTION: Due to the relaxing effect of the oil, marjoram should not be used before driving or doing anything that requires full attention. In large amounts, marjoram can be stupefying on the mind.

Myrtle

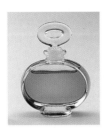

Botanical Name: *Myrtus communis*
Family: *Myrtaceae*
The essential oil is extracted from the leaves, twigs, and flowering tops of the shrub.
Scent of the oil: Fresh, camphorous, vaporous
Plant Description: Myrtle is an evergreen shrub that grows to a height of about 10–18 feet (3–5.5 meters), and has scented dark green leaves and small fragrant white flowers with many yellow stamens, followed by edible bluish-black berries.

AROMATHERAPY USES

Calming; the vapors open sinus and breathing passages; mood uplifting, refreshing; helpful for meditation; relieves pain.

Neroli

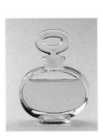

Botanical Name: *Citrus aurantium*
Family: *Rutaceae*
The essential oil is extracted from the blossoms of the tree.
Scent of the oil: Sweet, floral, citrus
Plant Description: Bitter orange is an evergreen citrus tree that grows to a height of about 20–30 feet (6–9 meters), and has fragrant white flowers that yield neroli oil.

AROMATHERAPY USES

Calms nervous tension, relaxes hyperactive children; promotes a restful sleep; mood uplifting, boosts confidence, helps soothe emotional upsets; soothes the intestines; helps to relieve menstrual discomfort.

Orange (Bitter or Sweet)

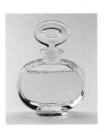

Botanical Name: *Citrus aurantium* (Bitter orange); *Citrus sinensis* (Sweet orange)
Family: *Rutaceae*
The essential oil is extracted from the peel of the fruit of the tree.
Scent of the oil: Fresh, sweet citrus
Plant Description: Orange is an evergreen citrus tree that grows to a

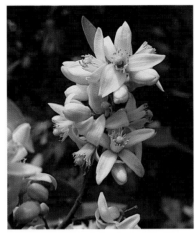

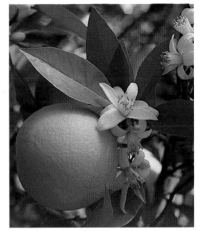

Neroli   *Orange*

height of about 20–30 feet (6–9 meters), and has fragrant white flowers that develop into edible orange-colored fruits.

AROMATHERAPY USES
Cooling; calming, reduces stress; promotes a restful sleep; mood uplifting, relieves emotional tension and stress, calms angry and irritable children; improves mental clarity and alertness; purifying, helps to reduce cellulite; relieves spasms.
PRECAUTION: Orange oil can irritate the skin and should either be avoided or used with extra care by people who have sensitive skin. Use small amounts. Orange is phototoxic. Avoid exposure to direct sunlight for several hours after applying the oil on the skin.

Patchouli

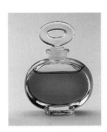

Botanical Name: *Pogostemon cablin, P. patchouli*
Family: *Lamiaceae*
The essential oil is extracted from the leaves of the plant.
Scent of the oil: Heavy, earthy
Plant Description: Patchouli is a plant that grows to a height of about 3 feet (0.9 meter), and has whorls of white flowers with colors of light purple or lavender.

AROMATHERAPY USES
Nerve stimulant; prevents sleep; mood uplifting, euphoric, aphrodisiac; repels insects; healing to the skin.

Peppermint

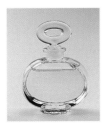

Botanical Name: *Mentha piperita*
Family: *Lamiaceae*
The essential oil is extracted from the whole plant.
Scent of the oil: Fresh, sweet mint, penetrating vapors

Plant Description: Peppermint is a plant that grows to a height of about 1–3 feet (0.3–0.9 meter), and has a purplish stem and pale violet flowers.

AROMATHERAPY USES

Cooling; the vapors open sinus and breathing passages; mood uplifting—especially for people who have a slow metabolism, refreshing, reviving, aphrodisiac; stimulates the brain, nerves, and metabolism; improves mental clarity, alertness, the ability to concentrate, and memory, sharpens the senses; encourages communication; helps to revive a person from a fainting spell or shock; increases physical strength and endurance; improves digestion, increases the appetite, relieves flatulence and nausea, sweetens the intestines, freshens bad breath; relieves pain, inflammation, menstrual pain, and cramps; reduces lactation; repels insects, kills parasites; soothes itching skin.

PRECAUTION: Peppermint oil can irritate the skin and should either be avoided or used with extra care by people who have sensitive skin. Use small amounts. It is best to avoid using the oil before bedtime due to the stimulating effect on the nervous system.

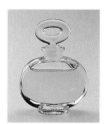

Pimento Berry (Allspice)

Botanical Name: *Pimenta dioica, P. officinalis*
Family: *Myrtaceae*
The essential oil is extracted from the dried unripe berries of the tree.
Scent of the oil: Warm, spicy, sweet, cinnamon-clove-like
Plant Description: Pimento is an evergreen tree that grows to a height of about 30–70 feet (9–21 meters), and has leathery leaves and small white flowers that develop into aromatic berries that turn dark brown when ripe.

AROMATHERAPY USES

Warming, improves circulation; calms the nerves, removes stress; promotes a restful sleep; the vapors open sinus and breathing passages; mood uplifting; improves digestion; purifying, helps to reduce cellulite; loosens tight muscles; lessens pain.

PRECAUTION: Pimento berry oil can irritate the skin and should either be avoided or used with extra care by people with sensitive skin.

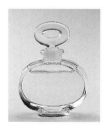

Ravensara Aromatica

Botanical Name: *Cinnamomum camphora, Ravensara aromatica*
Family: *Lauraceae*
The essential oil is extracted from the leaves of the havozo tree.
Scent of the oil: Camphorous, penetrating vapors
Plant Description: Havozo is a small tree.

Calming; reduces stress; the vapors open sinus and breathing passages; mood uplifting, refreshing; improves mental clarity; relieves aches and pains.

Rose

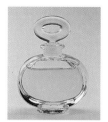

Botanical Name: *Rosa centifolia, R. damascena*
Family: *Rosaceae*
The essential oil is extracted from the flowers of the bush.
Scent of the oil: Sweet floral
Plant Description: There are many varieties of the rose bush that grow to various heights and produce sweet, fragrant flowers.

AROMATHERAPY USES

Cooling; calming, reduces stress, calms emotional shock and grief; mood uplifting, aphrodisiac; purifying; lessens aches, pains, and inflammation; balances the female hormonal and reproductive system; regenerates the skin cells, especially beneficial for dry, sensitive, inflamed, red, aging skin.

Rosemary

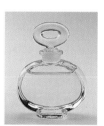

Botanical Name: *Rosmarinus officinalis*
Family: *Lamiaceae*
The essential oil is extracted from the flowers and leaves of the shrub.
Scent of the oil: Camphorous, penetrating vapors
Plant Description: Rosemary is an aromatic evergreen bushy shrub that grows to a height of about 2–6 feet (0.6–2 meters), and has leathery needle-shaped leaves and small blue flowers.

AROMATHERAPY USES

Warming, improves circulation; the vapors open sinus and breathing passages; mood uplifting—especially for people who have a slow metab-

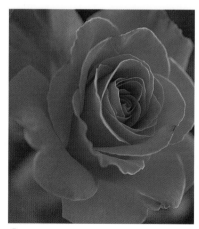

Rose

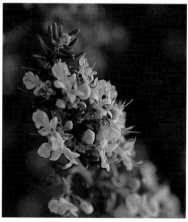

Rosemary

olism, refreshing; stimulates the heart, nerves, adrenal glands, metabolism, and all other body functions; improves mental clarity, alertness, and the memory; improves the digestion; purifying, helps to eliminate cellulite and lymphatic deposits from the body; relieves aches and pains; disinfectant; repels insects.

PRECAUTION: Rosemary should not be used by people prone to epileptic seizures. It is best to avoid using the oil before bedtime due to the stimulating effect.

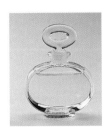

Sage (Spanish)
Botanical Name: *Salvia lavandulifolia*
Family: *Lamiaceae*
The essential oil is extracted from the flowers and leaves of the plant.
Scent of the oil: Camphorous, penetrating vapors
Plant Description: Sage is an evergreen plant that grows to a height of about 2½ feet (0.76 meter), and has small purple flowers.

AROMATHERAPY USES
Improves circulation; reduces stress; improves alertness; improves digestion; purifying, helps to reduce cellulite; relaxes sore muscles; lessens aches, pains, and menstrual pain; strengthening to the body; suppresses perspiration and lactation.

PRECAUTION: Spanish sage is less toxic and safer to use than common sage. Neither sage should be used by people prone to epileptic seizures.

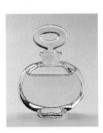

Sandalwood
Botanical Name: *Santalum album*
Family: *Santalaceae*
The essential oil is extracted from the inner wood of the tree.
Scent of the oil: Sweet, woody
Plant Description: Sandalwood is an evergreen tree that grows to a height of about 30 feet (9 meters), and has small pale yellow to purple flowers and small dark fruits containing a seed.

AROMATHERAPY USES
Calming, relaxing, reduces stress; promotes a restful sleep; encourages dreaming; soothing to the breathing passages; mood uplifting, euphoric, aphrodisiac; brings out emotions; helpful for meditation; healing and moisturizing to the skin; used as a fixative to hold the scent of a fragrance.

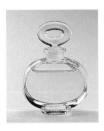

Spearmint
Botanical Name: *Mentha spicata, M. viridis*
Family: *Lamiaceae*
The essential oil is extracted from the leaves and flowering tops of the plant.

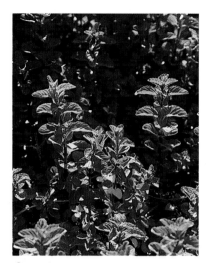

Spearmint

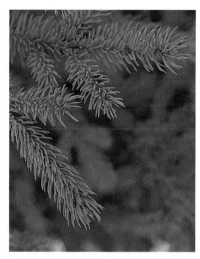

Spruce

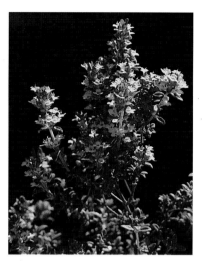

Thyme

Scent of the oil: Fresh, sweet mint, penetrating vapors
Plant Description: Spearmint is a plant that grows to a height of about 1–3 feet (0.3–0.9 meter), and has shiny bright green leaves and white or lilac flowers.

AROMATHERAPY USES
Cooling; the vapors open sinus and breathing passages; mood uplifting, refreshing, reviving, aphrodisiac; stimulates and strengthens the nerves, stimulates the metabolism, increases physical strength and endurance; improves mental clarity, alertness, ability to concentrate, and the memory, sharpens the senses; encourages communication; improves digestion, increases the appetite, relieves flatulence, freshens the breath and the intestines; relieves aches, pains, inflammation, and menstrual pain; repels insects; soothes itching skin.
PRECAUTION: Spearmint oil can irritate the skin and should either be avoided or used with extra care by people who have sensitive skin. Use small amounts. It is best to avoid using the oil before bedtime due to the stimulating effect on the nervous system.

Spikenard

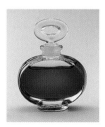

Botanical Name: *Nardostachys jatamansi*
Family: *Valerianaceae*
The essential oil is extracted from the roots of the plant.
Scent of the oil: Sweet, earthy
Plant Description: Spikenard is an aromatic plant that grows to a height of about 2 feet (0.6 meter), and has pink bell-shaped flowers.

AROMATHERAPY USES
Calming, relaxing, reduces stress; promotes a restful sleep; mood uplifting; reduces inflammation.

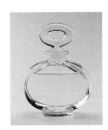

Spruce

Botanical Name: *Picea mariana*
Family: *Pinaceae*
The essential oil is extracted from the bark and branches of the tree.
Scent of the oil: Fresh, sweet, turpentine-like, vaporous
Plant Description: Spruce is an evergreen tree that grows to a height ranging from 70 to 200 feet (21–61 meters), and has bluish-green needle-like leaves, purple flowers, and purple male and female cones maturing to a brownish color.

AROMATHERAPY USES
Calming, reduces stress; the vapors open sinus and breathing passages; mood uplifting, euphoric; improves mental clarity; brings out inner feelings and encourages communication; disinfectant.

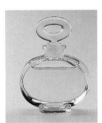

Tangerine

Botanical Name: *Citrus reticulata*
Family: *Rutaceae*
The essential oil is extracted from the peel of the fruit of the tree.
Scent of the oil: Sweet citrus
Plant Description: Tangerine is an evergreen citrus tree that grows to a height of about 20–25 feet (6–7.6 meters), and has fragrant white flowers that develop into edible orange-colored fruits.

AROMATHERAPY USES
Cooling; calming, relieves emotional tension and stress, calms angry and irritable children; promotes a restful sleep; mood uplifting; improves mental clarity and alertness, sharpens the mind; purifying, helps to reduce cellulite.
PRECAUTION: Tangerine oil can irritate the skin and should either be avoided or used with extra care by people who have sensitive skin. Use small amounts. Tangerine is phototoxic. Avoid exposure to direct sunlight for several hours after applying the oil on the skin.

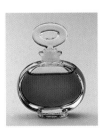

Thyme

Botanical Name: *Thymus aestivus, T. ilerdensis, T. valentianus, T. vulgaris* (Red Thyme); *T. webbianus* (Common Thyme); *T. satureiodes, T. vulgaris var. linalol* (Sweet Thyme); *T. citriodorus* (Lemon Thyme).
Family: *Lamiaceae*
The essential oil is extracted from the leaves and flowering tops of the plant.
Scent of the oil: Warm, sharp, spicy, herbaceous. The variety *Thymus citriodorus* has a lemony scent.
Plant Description: Thyme is an evergreen plant that grows to a height of about 1 foot (0.3 meter), and has small gray-green leaves and white, pink, or pale lilac flowers.

Heating, improves circulation; relaxes the nerves; the vapors open sinus and breathing passages; mood uplifting, stimulates the thyroid gland, increases physical endurance and energy; improves mental clarity and alertness, sharpens the senses; improves digestion, cleanses the intestines; purifying, helps to eliminate cellulite, waste material and excessive fluids from the body; relieves aches, pains, inflammation, and spasms; induces perspiration; disinfectant; repels insects, kills lice.

Comments: The varieties *Thymus citriodorus, T. satureiodes,* and *T. vulgaris var. linalol* are less irritating to the skin and less toxic than common thyme.

PRECAUTION: Thyme oil can irritate the skin and should either be avoided or used with extra care by people who have sensitive skin. Use small amounts. Thyme should not be used by people prone to epileptic seizures.

Vanilla

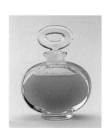

Botanical Name: *Vanilla fragrans, V. planifolia*
Family: *Orchidaceae*
The essential oil is extracted from the unripe pods of the plant.
Scent of the oil: Richly sweet, smokey
Plant Description: Vanilla is a climbing plant that reaches a height of about 12 feet (3.6 meters), and has clusters of pale yellow-green flowers followed by green pods containing many small seeds.

AROMATHERAPY USES

Calming, reduces stress; promotes a restful sleep; encourages dreaming; mood uplifting, aphrodisiac.

Comments: In the formulas given in this book, it is recommended that the vanilla CO_2 extracted oil be used.

Ylang-Ylang

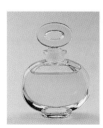

Botanical Name: *Cananga odorata var. genuina*
Family: *Annonaceae*
The essential oil is extracted from the flowers of the tree.
Scent of the oil: Heavy sweet, floral
Plant Description: Ylang-Ylang is an evergreen tree that grows to a height of about 100 feet (30 meters), and has glossy leaves and large yellow fragrant flowers.

AROMATHERAPY USES

Calming, relaxing, reduces stress; promotes a restful sleep; mood uplifting, euphoric, aphrodisiac; brings out feelings, enhances communication; loosens tight muscles; lessens pain; disinfectant.

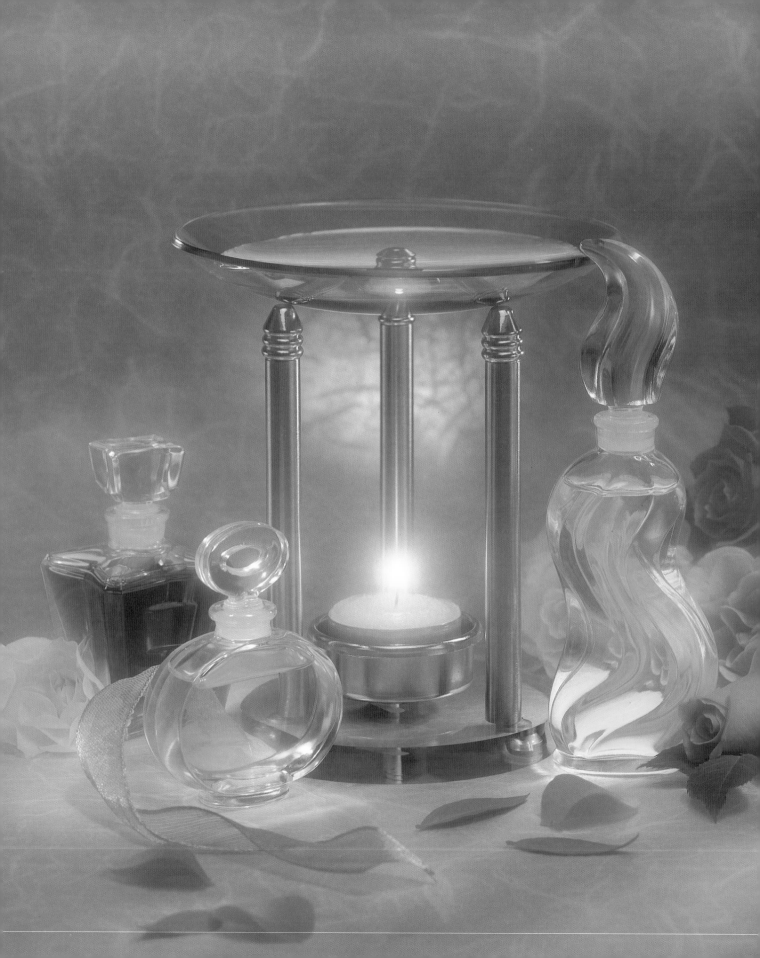

Chapter 7
Preparing Your Own Aromatic Blends

Over the past 50 years our dependency on the use of chemicals as ingredients in products has proliferated in practically every facet of our life. It is commonplace today for a person to be exposed to thousands of chemicals daily—some very harmful to health.

It is becoming more obvious to many people that we must take more responsibility for our actions and use products that are compatible with our natural environment. Our earth is a sacred embodiment that makes all life possible. We have an obligation to preserve and maintain her integrity for not only the benefit of our future, but future generations as well.

The essential oils can be combined together to produce the finest, most effective formulas to improve the quality of life, and, at the same time, be safe and compatible with our environment.

Before blending and using any of these formulas, please carefully read Chapter 3.

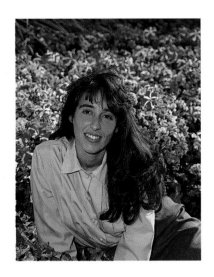

Enjoying Life More

We often are faced with so many demands, responsibilities, and obligations that sometimes we lose ourselves in the midst of trying to keep up. Life is too short to let the days rush by without experiencing the simple pleasures that are so worthwhile and beautiful. So set aside time today and enjoy nature; luxuriate in a soothing warm scented bath; indulge in a nurturing and stress-relieving massage; or spend a quiet evening at home with someone special and enjoy a dinner by candlelight with a wonderful mood-uplifting fragrance vaporizing from an aroma lamp. Don't let another day pass without enjoying life to the fullest.

Baths

Select one of the bath formulas. Mix the oils together in a small glass bottle. Fill the bathtub with water as warm as you like and pour the blend into the bathwater. Distribute the oils evenly throughout the tub. For the formulas that require bath salts, dissolve the salt well into the water to prevent it from settling on the bottom of the tub. Enter the bath immediately and relax for thirty minutes.

Aching Muscles—Bath

Lavender	5 drops	Chamomile (Roman)	4 drops
Manuka	4 drops	Rosemary	4 drops
Gingergrass	4 drops	Guaiacwood	4 drops
Ravensara Aromatica	2 drops	Litsea Cubeba	3 drops
Carrier Oil	1 teaspoon (5 ml)	Carrier Oil	1 teaspoon (5 ml)
Sea Salt	1 cup/8 ounces (226.8 gm)	Sea Salt	1 cup/8 ounces (226.8 gm)

֎ ֎

Lavender	5 drops	Manuka	4 drops
Myrtle	4 drops	Lavender	4 drops
Havozo Bark	3 drops	Sage (Spanish)	3 drops
Gingergrass	3 drops	Orange	3 drops
Carrier Oil	1 teaspoon (5 ml)	Carrier Oil	1 teaspoon (5 ml)
Sea Salt	1 cup/8 ounces (226.8 gm)	Sea Salt	1 cup/8 ounces (226.8 gm)

֎ ֎

Rejuvenate—Bath

Hyssop Decumbens	4 drops	Rosemary	4 drops
Gingergrass	3 drops	Fir Needles	4 drops
Helichrysum	3 drops	Hyssop Decumbens	3 drops
Rosemary	3 drops	Spearmint	3 drops
Lime	2 drops	Patchouli	1 drop
Carrier Oil	1 teaspoon (5 ml)	Carrier Oil	1 teaspoon (5 ml)
Sea Salt	1 cup/8 ounces (226.8 gm)	Sea Salt	1 cup/8 ounces (226.8 gm)

Sensual—Bath

Neroli	4 drops	Lime	4 drops
Vanilla	4 drops	Rose	3 drops
Manuka	3 drops	Ylang-Ylang	3 drops
Patchouli	3 drops	Gingergrass	3 drops
Carrier Oil	1 teaspoon (5 ml)	Carrier Oil	1 teaspoon (5 ml)
Amyris	4 drops	Havozo Bark	4 drops
Manuka	4 drops	Orange	4 drops
Vanilla	3 drops	Ylang-Ylang	3 drops
Cabreuva	2 drops	Ambrette Seed	3 drops
Carrier Oil	1 teaspoon (5 ml)	Carrier Oil	1 teaspoon (5 ml)

Tranquillity—Bath

Chamomile (Roman)	4 drops	Spruce	4 drops
Neroli	4 drops	Tangerine	4 drops
Spikenard	4 drops	Myrtle	3 drops
Juniper Berry	3 drops	Clary Sage	3 drops
Carrier Oil	1 teaspoon (5 ml)	Carrier Oil	1 teaspoon (5 ml)
Lavender	4 drops	Spikenard	4 drops
Lemon	4 drops	Chamomile (Roman)	4 drops
Copaiba	4 drops	Ylang-Ylang	4 drops
Manuka	3 drops	Vanilla	2 drops
Carrier Oil	1 teaspoon (5 ml)	Carrier Oil	1 teaspoon (5 ml)

Be the Best You Can Be

It is unfortunate that there are people who possess phenomenal skills, talents, and valuable knowledge but make little or no use of these great attributes. It is so important to utilize all that we have, to make a better and more meaningful life for ourselves and the people we care for—and to develop to nothing less than our fullest potential.

Select one of the *Be the Best You Can Be* application, diffuser, inhaler, or mist spray formulas. Find a quiet, comfortable place to relax where you will not be disturbed, play soft music (optional), and use the formula. Close your eyes and spend about 20–30 minutes pondering the skills, talents, and knowledge you possess that you haven't been utilizing to the fullest. List them on the *Be the Best You Can Be Worksheet*. After taking action with this important insight, complete the rest of the worksheet. Repeat this exercise until good results are obtained.

Be the Best You Can Be—Application
Apply one of these formulas to the wrists, upper chest, and back of the neck until the oil is fully absorbed into the skin. Breathe the vapors in deeply.

Tangerine	4 drops	Sandalwood		4 drops
Gingergrass	3 drops	Rose		3 drops
Neroli	3 drops	Pimento Berry		3 drops
Carrier Oil	2 teaspoons (10 ml)	Carrier Oil	2 teaspoons (10 ml)	

Guaiacwood	5 drops	Myrtle		3 drops
Spearmint	3 drops	Spruce		3 drops
Litsea Cubeba	2 drops	Vanilla		3 drops
Carrier Oil	2 teaspoons (10 ml)	Cedarwood (Atlas)		1 drop
		Carrier Oil	2 teaspoons (10 ml)	

Be the Best You Can Be—Diffuser
Choose one of these formulas. Place the essential oils in the designated container of the diffuser, then turn on the unit to disperse the aroma into the air.

Orange	40%	Spearmint	40%
Grapefruit	30%	Orange	30%
Litsea Cubeba	20%	Spruce	20%
Clove Bud	10%	Clary Sage	10%

Tangerine	40%	Spearmint	60%
Spruce	40%	Litsea Cubeba	20%
Gingergrass	10%	Havozo Bark	20%
Thyme	10%		

Be the Best You Can Be—Inhaler
Choose one of these formulas. Combine the essential oils into a small glass bottle with a wide opening. Inhale the vapors slowly and deeply. Then tightly cap the bottle after using.

*Be the Best You Can Be Worksheet**

Date: _____

SKILLS, TALENTS, AND KNOWLEDGE I HAVE THAT I HAVEN'T BEEN UTILIZING TO THE FULLEST:

1. _____
2. _____
3. _____
4. _____
5. _____
6. _____

ACTION PLAN—
STEPS I NEED TO TAKE IN ORDER TO REACH MY FULL POTENTIAL:

1. _____
2. _____
3. _____
4. _____
5. _____
6. _____

RESULTS
AFTER 3 MONTHS OF PUTTING ACTIONS INTO PRACTICE:

Date: _____
1. _____
2. _____
3. _____
4. _____
5. _____
6. _____

CONCLUSION:

_____
_____
_____
_____
_____
_____

Please make a copy of this worksheet and fill it out.

❂		❂	
Orange	15 drops	Vanilla	15 drops
Sandalwood	7 drops	Neroli	5 drops
Pimento Berry	5 drops	Litsea Cubeba	5 drops
Rose	3 drops	Amyris	5 drops

❂		❂	
Guaiacwood	10 drops	Spearmint	10 drops
Manuka	8 drops	Vanilla	10 drops
Spearmint	8 drops	Havozo Bark	7 drops
Gingergrass	4 drops	Patchouli	3 drops

Be the Best You Can Be—Mist Spray

Choose one of these formulas. Fill a fine-mist spray bottle with four ounces (120 ml) of purified water, add the essential oils, tightly cap the bottle, and shake well. Mist numerous times over the head with eyes closed. Breathe the vapors in deeply.

❂		❂	
Orange	65 drops	Lemon	80 drops
Lemon	45 drops	Vanilla	40 drops
Rose	20 drops	Neroli	20 drops
Guaiacwood	10 drops	Guaiacwood	10 drops
Cassia Bark	5 drops	Pure Water	4 ounces (120 ml)
Pure Water	4 ounces (120 ml)		

❂		❂	
Tangerine	60 drops	Spearmint	75 drops
Grapefruit	30 drops	Spruce	40 drops
Hyssop Decumbens	20 drops	Havozo Bark	30 drops
Clove Bud	20 drops	Copaiba	5 drops
Gingergrass	20 drops	Pure Water	4 ounces (120 ml)
Pure Water	4 ounces (120 ml)		

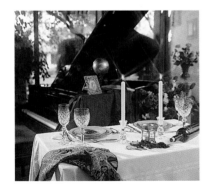

Candlelight Dinner

Create a delightful ambience using the aromatic oils to turn your dinner engagement into a special occasion. The aromas can reduce stress, uplift your mood, and help you have an enjoyable time.

Candlelight Dinner—Aroma Lamp

Place the aroma lamp on your dining-room table. Select one of these formulas and, when dinner is served, fill the container with water, add the essential oils, and heat. Play soft music, light the candles, dim the lights, and enjoy a wonderful evening.

❂ ❂

Lemon	7 drops	Fir Needles	8 drops
Lime	7 drops	Spruce	8 drops
Pimento Berry	7 drops	Orange	5 drops
Amyris	4 drops	Guaiacwood	4 drops

Tangerine	7 drops	Spearmint	15 drops
Gingergrass	7 drops	Patchouli	5 drops
Lime	6 drops	Cassia Bark	5 drops
Cassia Bark	5 drops		

Spruce	7 drops	Peppermint	10 drops
Litsea Cubeba	6 drops	Spruce	10 drops
Spearmint	6 drops	Spearmint	5 drops
Amyris	6 drops		

Candlelight Dinner—Diffuser

Select one of these formulas. Place the essential oils in the designated container of the diffuser, then turn on the unit to disperse the aroma into the air.

Orange	50%	Spearmint	40%
Spruce	30%	Orange	40%
Pimento Berry	10%	Fennel (Sweet)	20%
Cassia Bark	10%		

Fir Needles	40%	Tangerine	40%
Spruce	30%	Litsea Cubeba	30%
Tangerine	30%	Geranium	20%
		Cassia Bark	10%

Litsea Cubeba	30%	Gingergrass	40%
Gingergrass	30%	Spruce	40%
Mandarin	30%	Spearmint	20%
Cassia Bark	10%		

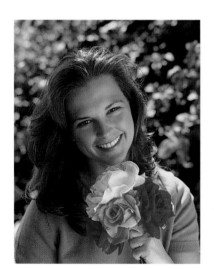

Choose To Be Happy

Some people seemingly have everything going for them—good looks, personality, intelligence, and talent—but yet they are not happy, while other people can make themselves happy with very little. Long-term happiness comes from deep within—it is a mind-set, an attitude reflecting our perceptions and the things we do to get satisfaction out of life. Once you've decided that you want to be happy, these formulas can enhance your mood.

Choose To Be Happy—Application

Apply one of these formulas to the upper chest and the back of the neck until the oil is fully absorbed into the skin. Breathe the vapors in deeply.

Litsea Cubeba	2 drops	Champaca Flower	2 drops
Vanilla	2 drops	Neroli	2 drops
Patchouli	1 drop	Amyris	1 drop
Carrier Oil	1 teaspoon (5 ml)	Carrier Oil	1 teaspoon (5 ml)

Neroli	3 drops	Spearmint	2 drops
Rose	1 drop	Havozo Bark	2 drops
Cedarwood (Atlas)	1 drop	Patchouli	1 drop
Carrier Oil	1 teaspoon (5 ml)	Carrier Oil	1 teaspoon (5 ml)

Rose	2 drops	Spearmint	2 drops
Champaca Flower	2 drops	Neroli	2 drops
Pimento Berry	1 drop	Spikenard	1 drop
Carrier Oil	1 teaspoon (5 ml)	Carrier Oil	1 teaspoon (5 ml)

Choose To Be Happy—Aroma Lamp

Select one of these formulas. Fill the container with water, add the essential oils, and heat. Breathe the vapors in deeply.

Vanilla	10 drops	Tangerine	15 drops
Spearmint	7 drops	Patchouli	5 drops
Spruce	7 drops	Vanilla	5 drops
Litsea Cubeba	6 drops	Cassia Bark	5 drops

Ylang-Ylang	15 drops	Orange	10 drops
Lime	10 drops	Grapefruit	10 drops
Clove Bud	5 drops	Chamomile (Roman)	7 drops
		Cassia Bark	3 drops

Choose To Be Happy—Diffuser

Select one of these formulas. Place the essential oils in the designated container of the diffuser, then turn on the unit to disperse the aroma into the air.

Orange	40%	Tangerine	50%
Spearmint	20%	Spruce	30%
Cinnamon Leaf	20%	Fir Needles	20%
Gingergrass	20%		

Chamomile (Roman)	50%	Spearmint	30%
Orange	20%	Chamomile (Roman)	30%
Lime	20%	Mandarin	30%
Cassia Bark	10%	Pimento Berry	10%

Choose To Be Happy—Inhaler

Select one of these formulas. Combine the essential oils into a small glass bottle with a wide opening. Inhale the vapors slowly and deeply. Then tightly cap the bottle and use again whenever necessary.

Mandarin	15 drops	Spearmint	10 drops
Chamomile (Roman)	5 drops	Cinnamon Leaf	6 drops
Vanilla	5 drops	Sandalwood	5 drops
		Spruce	4 drops

Tangerine	15 drops	Litsea Cubeba	10 drops
Guaiacwood	5 drops	Vanilla	10 drops
Neroli	5 drops	Patchouli	5 drops

Orange	10 drops	Rose	10 drops
Helichrysum	5 drops	Sandalwood	7 drops
Hyssop Decumbens	5 drops	Clove Bud	5 drops
Neroli	5 drops	Lavender	3 drops

Choose To Be Happy—Mist Spray

Select one of these formulas. Fill a fine-mist spray bottle with four ounces (120 ml) of purified water, add the essential oils, tighten the cap, and shake well. Mist numerous times over the head with eyes closed. Breathe the vapors in deeply.

Tangerine	70 drops	Spearmint	50 drops
Lemon	30 drops	Gingergrass	30 drops
Litsea Cubeba	20 drops	Eucalyptus Citriodora	20 drops
Neroli	20 drops	Cinnamon Leaf	20 drops
Guaiacwood	10 drops	Peppermint	20 drops
Pure Water	4 ounces (120 ml)	Grapefruit	10 drops
		Pure Water	4 ounces (120 ml)

Orange	60 drops	Tangerine	50 drops
Helichyrsum	30 drops	Lemon	50 drops
Neroli	25 drops	Spearmint	25 drops
Copaiba	20 drops	Vanilla	15 drops
Hyssop Decumbens	15 drops	Patchouli	10 drops
Pure Water	4 ounces (120 ml)	Pure Water	4 ounces (120 ml)

Lime	50 drops	Grapefruit	60 drops
Orange	50 drops	Gingergrass	25 drops
Chamomile (Roman)	20 drops	Chamomile (Roman)	25 drops
Neroli	15 drops	Cedarwood (Atlas)	20 drops
Patchouli	15 drops	Vanilla	20 drops
Pure Water	4 ounces (120 ml)	Pure Water	4 ounces (120 ml)

Communicate Effectively

Proper communication is a great tool to prevent or solve problems and disagreements between people. But there are times when we are extremely hurt or offended due to what someone has done to us. At that point our communication may turn into an attack instrument to hurt the other individual. When in a situation such as this, select and use one of the *Communicate Effectively* application or mist spray formulas to relax and help dissipate the hurt. Then fill out the *Communicate Effectively Worksheet* to help you rethink how to present your point of view politely and most effectively to minimize the conflict and make peace. For best results, you may need to practice this exercise several times.

Communicate Effectively—Application

Apply one of these formulas to the upper chest and the back of the neck until the oil is fully absorbed into the skin. Breathe the vapors in deeply.

Spruce	3 drops	Chamomile (Roman)	4 drops
Tangerine	3 drops	Orange	3 drops
Cedarwood (Atlas)	2 drops	Juniper Berry	3 drops
Vanilla	2 drops	Carrier Oil	2 teaspoons (10 ml)
Carrier Oil	2 teaspoons (10 ml)		

Lime	5 drops	Lime	4 drops
Vanilla	3 drops	Cabreuva	3 drops
Copaiba	2 drops	Pimento Berry	3 drops
Carrier Oil	2 teaspoons (10 ml)	Carrier Oil	2 teaspoons (10 ml)

Cedarwood (Atlas)	4 drops	Spruce	3 drops
Spruce	3 drops	Grapefruit	3 drops
Litsea Cubeba	3 drops	Gingergrass	2 drops
Carrier Oil	2 teaspoons (10 ml)	Copaiba	2 drops
		Carrier Oil	2 teaspoons (10 ml)

Communicate Effectively—Mist Spray

Choose one of these formulas. Fill a fine-mist spray bottle with four ounces (120 ml) of purified water, add the essential oils, tighten the cap, and shake well. Mist numerous times over the head with eyes closed. Breathe the vapors in deeply.

Spruce	40 drops	Litsea Cubeba	40 drops
Orange	40 drops	Orange	40 drops
Chamomile (Roman)	30 drops	Spearmint	30 drops
Cedarwood (Atlas)	30 drops	Manuka	20 drops
Vanilla	10 drops	Gingergrass	20 drops
Pure Water	4 ounces (120 ml)	Pure Water	4 ounces (120 ml)

Communicate Effectively Worksheet*

Date: _____

I FEEL ANGRY OR HURT BECAUSE:

_____
_____
_____
_____
_____

TO RESOLVE THE CONFLICT AND MAKE PEACE, I WANT TO POLITELY EXPLAIN MY POINT OF VIEW IN THESE WORDS:

_____
_____
_____
_____
_____
_____
_____
_____
_____
_____
_____

RESULTS AFTER THE COMMUNICATION:

Date: _____
_____
_____
_____
_____

CONCLUSION: 1 MONTH LATER

Date: _____
_____
_____
_____
_____

Please make a copy of this sheet and fill it out.

Lime	50 drops		Orange	50 drops
Fir Needles	40 drops		Lime	40 drops
Cinnamon Leaf	20 drops		Pimento Berry	20 drops
Vanilla	20 drops		Spearmint	20 drops
Copaiba	20 drops		Cabreuva	20 drops
Pure Water	4 ounces (120 ml)		Pure Water	4 ounces (120 ml)

❧

Gingergrass	50 drops		Chamomile (Roman)	40 drops
Orange	50 drops		Copaiba	40 drops
Copaiba	25 drops		Vanilla	20 drops
Vanilla	25 drops		Litsea Cubeba	20 drops
Pure Water	4 ounces (120 ml)		Havozo Bark	20 drops
			Cassia Bark	10 drops
			Pure Water	4 ounces (120 ml)

Dreams

Dreams are the windows of our subconscious mind, providing us with hidden messages and invaluable insights and information for what we need to know, learn, and accomplish.

Dreams—Application

Apply one of these formulas to the upper chest and back of the neck until the oil is fully absorbed into the skin.

Use before going to sleep. If you do not dream the first night, repeat application the following nights. For some people it may take several applications before obtaining desired results.

❧

Lavender	4 drops		Clary Sage	3 drops
Neroli	3 drops		Cabreuva	3 drops
Helichrysum	3 drops		Cinnamon Leaf	2 drops
Carrier Oil	2 teaspoons (10 ml)		Vanilla	2 drops
			Carrier Oil	2 teaspoons (10 ml)

❧

Helichrysum	3 drops		Vanilla	4 drops
Cinnamon Leaf	3 drops		Havozo Bark	3 drops
Tangerine	3 drops		Cinnamon Leaf	3 drops
Rosemary	1 drop		Carrier Oil	2 teaspoons (10 ml)
Carrier Oil	2 teaspoons (10 ml)			

❧

Orange	3 drops		Neroli	3 drops
Vanilla	3 drops		Cabreuva	3 drops
Chamomile (Roman)	2 drops		Mandarin	2 drops
Sage (Spanish)	2 drops		Vanilla	2 drops
Carrier Oil	2 teaspoons (10 ml)		Carrier Oil	2 teaspoons (10 ml)

Express Appreciation

We often go through life not clearly communicating to people how much we appreciate them and the good they do for us. Now we can take this extraordinary opportunity to let the special people around us know exactly how we feel.

Select one of the *Express Appreciation* application, diffuser, inhaler, or mist spray formulas. Find a quiet, comfortable place to relax where you will not be disturbed, play soft music (optional), and spend 20–30 minutes thinking of the people to whom you would like to express your appreciation. Then fill out the *Express Appreciation Worksheet* and either phone, write, or communicate your appreciation in person to each of the people you have chosen.

Express Appreciation—Application

Apply one of these formulas to the upper chest and the back of the neck until the oil is fully absorbed into the skin. Breathe the vapors in deeply.

❁

Spruce	3 drops	Vanilla	3 drops
Ylang-Ylang	3 drops	Tangerine	3 drops
Cinnamon Leaf	2 drops	Cinnamon Leaf	2 drops
Vanilla	2 drops	Guaiacwood	2 drops
Carrier Oil	2 teaspoons (10 ml)	Carrier Oil	2 teaspoons (10 ml)

❁

Havozo Bark	4 drops	Spruce	4 drops
Orange	3 drops	Havozo Bark	3 drops
Ylang-Ylang	3 drops	Chamomile (Roman)	3 drops
Carrier Oil	2 teaspoons (10 ml)	Carrier Oil	2 teaspoons (10 ml)

Express Appreciation—Diffuser

Choose one of these formulas. Place the essential oils in the designated container of the diffuser, then turn on the unit to disperse the aroma into the air.

❁

Orange	50%	Spruce	40%
Fir Needles	30%	Chamomile (Roman)	30%
Havozo Bark	20%	Havozo Bark	30%

❁

Tangerine	40%	Spruce	40%
Cinnamon Leaf	20%	Ylang-Ylang	20%
Spearmint	20%	Chamomile (Roman)	20%
Lemon	20%	Geranium	20%

❁

Express Appreciation—Inhaler

Choose one of these formulas. Combine the essential oils in a small glass bottle with a wide opening. Inhale the vapors slowly and deeply. Then tightly cap the bottle after using.

Havozo Bark	10 drops	Tangerine	15 drops
Vanilla	10 drops	Geranium	10 drops
Chamomile (Roman)	10 drops	Spearmint	5 drops

Orange	15 drops	Spruce	12 drops
Lemon	10 drops	Havozo Bark	10 drops
Fennel (Sweet)	5 drops	Cinnamon Leaf	8 drops

Express Appreciation—Mist Spray

Choose one of these formulas. Fill a fine-mist spray bottle with four ounces (120 ml) of purified water, add the essential oils, tighten the cap, and shake well. Mist numerous times over the head with eyes closed. Breathe the vapors in deeply.

Chamomile (Roman)	40 drops	Orange	60 drops
Vanilla	40 drops	Grapefruit	40 drops
Grapefruit	30 drops	Lemon	20 drops
Cinnamon Leaf	25 drops	Spruce	20 drops
Geranium	15 drops	Guaiacwood	10 drops
Pure Water	4 ounces (120 ml)	Pure Water	4 ounces (120 ml)

Fir Needles	40 drops	Tangerine	50 drops
Havozo Bark	40 drops	Spruce	30 drops
Litsea Cubeba	30 drops	Gingergrass	20 drops
Geranium	20 drops	Chamomile (Roman)	20 drops
Vanilla	20 drops	Fennel (Sweet)	20 drops
Pure Water	4 ounces (120 ml)	Cassia Bark	10 drops
		Pure Water	4 ounces (120 ml)

Festivity Room Fragrancing

These room fragrances will help add to the festivity at a time when guests visit, or even to cheer you up when you're alone at home. Enjoy the fragrance!

Festivity Room Fragrancing—Aroma Lamp

Select one of these formulas. Fill the container with water, add the essential oils, and heat.

*Express Appreciation Worksheet**

Date: _____

NAMES OF PEOPLE I WOULD LIKE TO EXPRESS MY APPRECIATION TO:

1. _____
2. _____
3. _____
4. _____
5. _____
6. _____

I WOULD LIKE TO TELL EACH PERSON:

1. _____
2. _____
3. _____
4. _____
5. _____
6. _____

RESULTS AFTER EXPRESSING APPRECIATION TO EACH PERSON:

1. _____
2. _____
3. _____
4. _____
5. _____
6. _____

CONCLUSION:
I HAVE LEARNED THE FOLLOWING FROM THIS EXPERIENCE

_____
_____
_____
_____
_____
_____

*Please make a copy of this worksheet and fill it out.

Spearmint	13 drops	Litsea Cubeba	9 drops
Vanilla	6 drops	Orange	9 drops
Lime	6 drops	Vanilla	6 drops
Cassia Bark	5 drops	Grapefruit	6 drops
❂		❂	
Vanilla	8 drops	Vanilla	10 drops
Lemon	7 drops	Orange	8 drops
Gingergrass	7 drops	Clove Bud	7 drops
Cassia Bark	4 drops	Patchouli	5 drops
Peppermint	4 drops		
❂		❂	
Peppermint	15 drops	Lemon	9 drops
Spruce	8 drops	Gingergrass	8 drops
Eucalyptus Citriodora	4 drops	Orange	8 drops
Cassia Bark	3 drops	Sage (Spanish)	5 drops

Festivity Room Fragrancing—Diffuser

Select one of these formulas. Place the essential oils in the designated container of the diffuser, then turn on the unit to disperse the aroma into the air.

❂		❂	
Orange	50%	Fir Needles	25%
Lime	20%	Spruce	25%
Grapefruit	20%	Orange	25%
Cassia Bark	10%	Peppermint	25%
❂		❂	
Gingergrass	30%	Gingergrass	40%
Peppermint	30%	Tangerine	30%
Lemon	30%	Lime	30%
Cassia Bark	10%		

Festivity Room Fragrancing—Lightbulb Ring

Select one of these formulas. Place the lightbulb ring on top of a cool lightbulb and drop the oils carefully into the grove of the ring. Turn on the light and enjoy the scent.

❂		❂	
Spearmint	8 drops	Neroli	6 drops
Vanilla	7 drops	Lime	5 drops
		Vanilla	3 drops
		Champaca Flower	1 drop
❂		❂	
Ylang-Ylang	10 drops	Tangerine	13 drops
Gingergrass	4 drops	Amyris	2 drops
Cassia Bark	1 drop		

Festivity Room Fragrancing—Mist Spray

Select one of these formulas. Fill a fine-mist spray bottle with four ounces (120 ml) of purified water, add the essential oils, tighten the cap, and shake well. Mist numerous times into the air for everyone to enjoy.

❧

Spearmint	60 drops	Lime	40 drops
Orange	40 drops	Tangerine	40 drops
Cinnamon Leaf	20 drops	Fennel (Sweet)	20 drops
Vanilla	20 drops	Vanilla	20 drops
Patchouli	10 drops	Pimento Berry	15 drops
Pure Water	4 ounces (120 ml)	Amyris	15 drops
		Pure Water	4 ounces (120 ml)

❧

Spruce	40 drops	Spearmint	40 drops
Eucalyptus Citriodora	40 drops	Gingergrass	40 drops
Fir Needles	30 drops	Cedarwood (Atlas)	20 drops
Peppermint	30 drops	Rosemary	20 drops
Cassia Bark	10 drops	Vanilla	20 drops
Pure Water	4 ounces (120 ml)	Cassia Bark	10 drops
		Pure Water	4 ounces (120 ml)

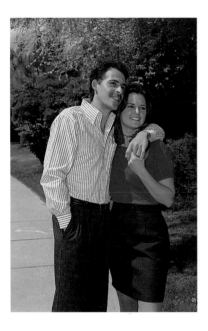

Get Closer to Someone You Love

With our fast-paced lifestyle and the daily struggle of trying to beat the clock to get everything done, we often neglect to spend quality time with the people we care for. Make it a priority to set aside time and give a massage to a loved one: son, daughter, brother, sister, spouse, friend, or anyone you'd like to get closer to, to open up a deeper relationship of caring, understanding, and communication.

Get Closer to Someone You Love—Massage

Massage one of these formulas into the back of the neck, shoulders, and back until the oil is fully absorbed into the skin. Breathe the vapors in deeply. Enjoy the time together.

❧

Orange	4 drops	Helichrysum	4 drops
Ambrette Seed	3 drops	Neroli	4 drops
Manuka	3 drops	Lime	4 drops
Neroli	3 drops	Sandalwood	3 drops
Spearmint	2 drops	Carrier Oil	1 tablespoon (15 ml)
Carrier Oil	1 tablespoon (15 ml)		

❧

Vanilla	6 drops		Tangerine	5 drops
Spruce	3 drops		Vanilla	4 drops
Guaiacwood	2 drops		Cypress	2 drops
Juniper Berry	2 drops		Cedarwood (Atlas)	2 drops
Fennel (Sweet)	2 drops		Spearmint	2 drops
Carrier Oil	1 tablespoon (15 ml)		Carrier Oil	1 tablespoon (15 ml)

❀

Vanilla	4 drops		Mandarin	5 drops
Orange	4 drops		Spikenard	4 drops
Gingergrass	3 drops		Gingergrass	3 drops
Pimento Berry	2 drops		Helichrysum	3 drops
Juniper Berry	2 drops		Carrier Oil	1 tablespoon (15 ml)
Carrier Oil	1 tablespoon (15 ml)			

Laziness Relief

Most people experience times when they feel sluggish, find it difficult to get going, and don't accomplish the work that needs to be done. Try one of the *Laziness Relief* diffuser, massage, or mist spray formulas to get a person out of a lazy state.

Laziness Relief—Diffuser

Select one of these formulas. Place the diffuser in the room where the work will be done. Put the essential oils in the designated container of the diffuser, then turn on the unit to disperse the aroma into the air.

❀

Spearmint	40%		Litsea Cubeba	30%
Hyssop Decumbens	30%		Peppermint	30%
Fennel (Sweet)	20%		Eucalyptus Citriodora	20%
Cassia Bark	10%		Cinnamon Leaf	20%

❀

Grapefruit	30%		Eucalyptus Citriodora	30%
Spearmint	30%		Rosemary	20%
Cinnamon Leaf	30%		Peppermint	20%
Thyme	10%		Grapefruit	20%
			Cassia Bark	10%

Laziness Relief—Massage

Massage one of these formulas to the upper chest and the back of the neck until the oil is fully absorbed into the skin. Breathe the vapors in deeply.

❀

Spearmint	4 drops		Peppermint	4 drops
Fennel (Sweet)	4 drops		Rosemary	4 drops
Patchouli	4 drops		Fennel (Sweet)	4 drops
Hyssop Decumbens	3 drops		Thyme	3 drops
Carrier Oil	1 tablespoon (15 ml)		Carrier Oil	1 tablespoon (15 ml)

Helichrysum	5 drops		Helichrysum	5 drops
Thyme	3 drops		Fennel (Sweet)	4 drops
Rosemary	3 drops		Lemon	3 drops
Gingergrass	2 drops		Thyme	3 drops
Patchouli	2 drops		Carrier Oil 1 tablespoon (15 ml)	
Carrier Oil 1 tablespoon (15 ml)				

Laziness Relief—Mist Spray

Select one of these formulas. Fill a fine-mist spray bottle with four ounces (120 ml) of purified water, add the essential oils, tighten the cap, and shake well. Mist numerous times over the head with eyes closed. Breathe the vapors in deeply.

Rosemary	50 drops		Peppermint	40 drops
Litsea Cubeba	40 drops		Gingergrass	40 drops
Lemon	20 drops		Fennel (Sweet)	30 drops
Spearmint	20 drops		Thyme	20 drops
Cassia Bark	10 drops		Eucalyptus Citriodora	20 drops
Cinnamon Leaf	10 drops		Pure Water 4 ounces (120 ml)	
Pure Water 4 ounces (120 ml)				

Grapefruit	40 drops		Grapefruit	50 drops
Spearmint	40 drops		Cinnamon Leaf	35 drops
Hyssop Decumbens	30 drops		Rose	30 drops
Helichrysum	20 drops		Lemon	30 drops
Thyme	20 drops		Vanilla	15 drops
Pure Water 4 ounces (120 ml)			Pure Water 4 ounces (120 ml)	

Make a Difference

All of us would like to see the world we live in become a better place. One good person can truly make a big difference in the lives of others. Think back when you were younger and how a good person was a positive influence on your life. Think of how important this person was to you and all the good memories you have. Now you can play the same meaningful role with other people in your life who need positive guidance. This could turn out to be the greatest gift you'll ever give.

Select one of the *Make a Difference* application, diffuser, inhaler, or mist spray formulas. Find a quiet, comfortable place to relax where you will not be disturbed, play soft music (optional), and use the formula. Close your eyes, reflect back, and think of the fond memories you have of a person who was a great influence in your life. Spend some time and capture these wonderful feelings. Afterward, think about the people in your life now who can benefit greatly from your guidance. Use the *Make a Difference Worksheet* to better organize your thoughts.

Make a Difference—Application

Apply one of these formulas to the upper chest and the back of the neck until the oil is fully absorbed into the skin. Breathe the vapors in deeply.

❀

Peppermint	4 drops	Spruce	3 drops
Vanilla	4 drops	Vanilla	3 drops
Thyme	2 drops	Cedarwood (Atlas)	2 drops
Carrier Oil	2 teaspoons (10 ml)	Fir Needles	2 drops
		Carrier Oil	2 teaspoons (10 ml)

❀

Orange	5 drops	Vanilla	4 drops
Chamomile (Roman)	3 drops	Rose	3 drops
Pimento Berry	2 drops	Gingergrass	3 drops
Carrier Oil	2 teaspoons (10 ml)	Carrier Oil	2 teaspoons (10 ml)

❀

Vanilla	4 drops	Orange	4 drops
Lime	3 drops	Chamomile (Roman)	2 drops
Peppermint	2 drops	Spruce	2 drops
Cedarwood (Atlas)	1 drop	Havozo Bark	2 drops
Carrier Oil	2 teaspoons (10 ml)	Carrier Oil	2 teaspoons (10 ml)

Make a Difference—Diffuser

Choose one of these formulas. Place the essential oils in the designated container of the diffuser, then turn on the unit to disperse the aroma into the air.

❀

Fir Needles	40%	Fir Needles	30%
Spearmint	20%	Orange	30%
Lime	20%	Pimento Berry	20%
Gingergrass	20%	Lime	20%

❀

Orange	40%	Peppermint	30%
Spruce	30%	Orange	20%
Grapefruit	20%	Fir Needles	20%
Havozo Bark	10%	Chamomile (Roman)	20%
		Thyme	10%

Make a Difference—Inhaler

Choose one of these formulas. Combine the essential oils in a small glass bottle with a wide opening. Inhale the vapors slowly and deeply. Then tightly cap the bottle after using.

❀

Vanilla	15 drops	Vanilla	10 drops
Orange	10 drops	Lime	8 drops
Spruce	5 drops	Cedarwood (Atlas)	7 drops
		Fir Needles	5 drops

*Make a Difference Worksheet**

Date:_____

PEOPLE I CAN GIVE POSITIVE GUIDANCE TO:

1. _____
2. _____
3. _____
4. _____
5. _____
6. _____

PLAN OF ACTION FOR EACH PERSON:

1. _____
2. _____
3. _____
4. _____
5. _____
6. _____

RESULTS AFTER 3 WEEKS:

Date:_____
_____
_____
_____
_____
_____
_____
_____

CONCLUSION AFTER 3 MONTHS:

Date:_____
_____
_____
_____
_____
_____
_____

Please make a copy of this sheet and fill it out.

Vanilla	20 drops	Orange	15 drops
Rose	5 drops	Thyme	5 drops
Clove Bud	5 drops	Cedarwood (Atlas)	5 drops
		Guaiacwood	5 drops

Make a Difference—Mist Spray

Choose one of these formulas. Fill a fine-mist spray bottle with four ounces (120 ml) of purified water, add the essential oils, tighten the cap, and shake well. Mist numerous times over the head with eyes closed. Breathe the vapors in deeply.

Peppermint	40 drops	Spruce	35 drops
Orange	40 drops	Vanilla	35 drops
Gingergrass	30 drops	Lemon	30 drops
Clove Bud	20 drops	Grapefruit	25 drops
Lemon	20 drops	Juniper Berry	15 drops
Pure Water	4 ounces (120 ml)	Cassia Bark	10 drops
		Pure Water	4 ounces (120 ml)

Orange	40 drops	Spearmint	40 drops
Grapefruit	40 drops	Cedarwood (Atlas)	40 drops
Eucalyptus Citriodora	25 drops	Vanilla	30 drops
Spruce	25 drops	Thyme	20 drops
Patchouli	20 drops	Orange	20 drops
Pure Water	4 ounces (120 ml)	Pure Water	4 ounces (120 ml)

Morning Affirmation

When arising in the morning, take a few minutes out to get the day started right with a positive mind-set. Select and use one of the application or inhaler formulas and reflect on the morning affirmation.

Today is a very precious day. I am grateful for having enough food to eat, clothing to wear, a shelter to live in, and people and pets who love me. There are many individuals in this world who are not so fortunate as I am, who lack these vital necessities.

From this day forward, I will carry out my responsibilities to the very best of my ability and extend love, kindness, consideration, respect, and understanding to all living beings around me.

I will uphold high standards, values, and principles. The choices and decisions I make are based not only on wishful thinking but on reality and truth. I am willing to correct my beliefs or thinking should I find them to be faulty.

I will conduct myself with the utmost integrity. I take full responsibility for all my actions. Should I make mistakes, I will use them as learning experiences to help me grow wiser and improve the quality of my life.

Let this precious day not pass without my having acquired new beneficial knowledge and done kind deeds. I realize that every good deed I do for others not only benefits them but also helps me feel good about myself.

I will set a positive example and serve as a role model for others to follow. By being as good as I can be, I will do my share toward making this a better world.

I am now ready to do everything I can possibly do to make this a great day!

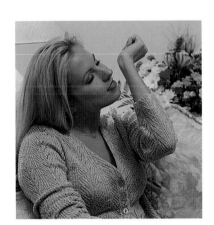

Morning Affirmation—Application

Apply one of these formulas to the wrists and/or to the upper chest and the back of the neck until the oil is fully absorbed into the skin. Breathe the vapors in deeply.

Spearmint	2 drops	Tangerine	1 drop
Vanilla	1 drop	Ambrette Seed	1 drop
Carrier Oil	½ teaspoon (2.5 ml)	Neroli	1 drop
		Carrier Oil	½ teaspoon (2.5 ml)

Neroli	1 drop	Rose	1 drop
Hyssop Decumbens	1 drop	Tangerine	1 drop
Helichrysum	1 drop	Vanilla	1 drop
Carrier Oil	½ teaspoon (2.5 ml)	Carrier Oil	½ teaspoon (2.5 ml)

Spearmint	2 drops	Spearmint	1 drop
Sandalwood	1 drop	Manuka	1 drop
Carrier Oil	½ teaspoon (2.5 ml)	Gingergrass	1 drop
		Carrier Oil	½ teaspoon (2.5 ml)

Morning Affirmation—Inhaler

Choose one of these formulas. Combine the essential oils into a small glass bottle with a wide opening. Inhale the vapors slowly and deeply. Then tightly cap the bottle after using.

Spearmint	12 drops	Tangerine	10 drops
Vanilla	4 drops	Rose	5 drops
Cassia Bark	4 drops	Vanilla	5 drops

Neroli	8 drops	Manuka	8 drops
Hyssop Decumbens	8 drops	Spearmint	8 drops
Helichrysum	4 drops	Gingergrass	4 drops

Vanilla	8 drops	Spearmint	10 drops
Ambrette Seed	4 drops	Sandalwood	10 drops
Clove Bud	4 drops		
Mandarin	4 drops		

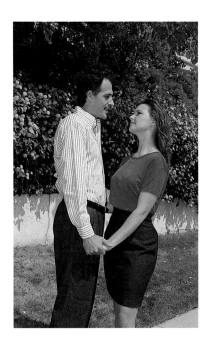

Open Your Heart for Love

Many of us have been close to relatives or friends and the relationships turned out to be very hurtful and caused great pain. As a result of these harmful experiences we may have closed off an important part that enables us to get close and love. If you feel ready now to release those hurt feelings and let them go, use one of these formulas and do the exercise.

Select one of the *Open Your Heart for Love* application, diffuser, inhaler, or mist spray formulas. Find a quiet, comfortable place to relax where you will not be disturbed, play soft music (optional), and use the formula. Close your eyes and spend 20–30 minutes thinking about the people and the hurtful feelings you want to let go of. Then fill out the *Open Your Heart for Love Worksheet*.

Open Your Heart for Love—Application

Apply one of these formulas to the wrists, upper chest, and the back of the neck until the oil is fully absorbed into the skin. Breathe the vapors in deeply.

Vanilla	3 drops	Orange	2 drops
Rose	2 drops	Rose	2 drops
Carrier Oil	1 teaspoon (5 ml)	Champaca Flower	1 drop
		Carrier Oil	1 teaspoon (5 ml)

Neroli	3 drops	Vanilla	3 drops
Ambrette Seed	2 drops	Champaca Flower	1 drop
Carrier Oil	1 teaspoon (5 ml)	Spruce	1 drop
		Carrier Oil	1 teaspoon (5 ml)

Open Your Heart for Love—Diffuser

Choose one of these formulas. Place the essential oils in the designated container of the diffuser, then turn on the unit to disperse the aroma into the air.

Tangerine	40%	Spruce	40%
Hyssop Decumbens	20%	Lime	30%
Manuka	20%	Havozo Bark	20%
Gingergrass	20%	Clove Bud	10%

Mandarin	30%	Orange	40%
Eucalyptus Citriodora	20%	Spruce	30%
Hyssop Decumbens	20%	Eucalyptus Citriodora	30%
Lavender	20%		
Cassia Bark	10%		

Open Your Heart for Love—Inhaler

Choose one of these formulas. Combine the essential oils in a small glass bottle with a wide opening. Inhale the vapors slowly and deeply. Then tightly cap the bottle after using.

◉		◉	
Vanilla	14 drops	Tangerine	13 drops
Rose	12 drops	Rose	10 drops
Cassia Bark	2 drops	Guaiacwood	7 drops
Lime	2 drops		

◉		◉	
Vanilla	13 drops	Neroli	16 drops
Spruce	10 drops	Guaiacwood	6 drops
Gingergrass	5 drops	Litsea Cubeba	5 drops
Marjoram	2 drops	Spearmint	3 drops

◉		◉	
Mandarin	15 drops	Havozo Bark	10 drops
Spruce	8 drops	Vanilla	10 drops
Lavender	4 drops	Gingergrass	5 drops
Guaiacwood	3 drops	Eucalyptus Citriodora	5 drops

Open Your Heart for Love—Mist Spray

Choose one of these formulas. Fill a fine-mist spray bottle with four ounces (120 ml) of purified water, add the essential oils, tighten the cap, and shake well. Mist numerous times over the head with eyes closed. Breathe the vapors in deeply.

◉		◉	
Ylang-Ylang	30 drops	Tangerine	50 drops
Helichrysum	30 drops	Vanilla	30 drops
Lemon	30 drops	Gingergrass	25 drops
Litsea Cubeba	30 drops	Spruce	15 drops
Cedarwood (Atlas)	20 drops	Guaiacwood	15 drops
Pimento Berry	10 drops	Lavender	10 drops
Pure Water	4 ounces (120 ml)	Cassia Bark	5 drops
		Pure Water	4 ounces (120 ml)

◉		◉	
Spearmint	60 drops	Tangerine	60 drops
Gingergrass	50 drops	Neroli	40 drops
Vanilla	30 drops	Vanilla	30 drops
Cedarwood (Atlas)	10 drops	Lemon	20 drops
Pure Water	4 ounces (120 ml)	Pure Water	4 ounces (120 ml)

Open Your Heart for Love Worksheet*

Date: _____

I AM NOW READY TO OPEN UP MY HEART FOR LOVE AND RELINQUISH MY
HURT AND PAINFUL FEELINGS FROM THE FOLLOWING PEOPLE:

Name: _____ Hurtful Feelings: _____

Name: _____ Hurtful Feelings: _____

Name: _____ Hurtful Feelings: _____

Name: _____ Hurtful Feelings: _____

Name: _____ Hurtful Feelings: _____

Name: _____ Hurtful Feelings: _____

1 MONTH LATER
CHANGES THAT HAVE OCCURRED IN MY LIFE DUE TO LETTING GO
OF MY HURTFUL FEELINGS:

Date: _____
_____
_____
_____
_____
_____

3 MONTH RESULTS:

Date: _____
_____
_____
_____
_____

OVERALL CONCLUSION:

_____
_____
_____
_____
_____
_____

Please make a copy of this worksheet and fill it out.

Peace and Calm

There are times when a person may want to be alone in a quiet atmosphere to comfort an overly stressed nervous system. Select one of the *Peace and Calm* application, inhaler, or mist spray formulas. Find a quiet, comfortable place to relax where you will not be disturbed, and enjoy the peacefulness.

Peace and Calm—Application

Apply one of these formulas to the upper chest, back of the neck, and shoulders until the oil is fully absorbed into the skin. Breathe the vapors in deeply.

Amyris	4 drops	Lemon	4 drops
Neroli	3 drops	Cypress	3 drops
Orange	3 drops	Tangerine	3 drops
Calophyllum	1 teaspoon (5 ml)	Calophyllum	1 teaspoon (5 ml)
Almond (Sweet)	1 teaspoon (5 ml)	Almond (Sweet)	1 teaspoon (5 ml)

Tangerine	4 drops	Tangerine	4 drops
Vanilla	3 drops	Marjoram	3 drops
Spikenard	3 drops	Amyris	3 drops
Calophyllum	1 teaspoon (5 ml)	Calophyllum	1 teaspoon (5 ml)
Almond (Sweet)	1 teaspoon (5 ml)	Almond (Sweet)	1 teaspoon (5 ml)

Peace and Calm—Inhaler

Choose one of these formulas. Combine the essential oils in a small glass bottle with a wide opening. Inhale the vapors slowly and deeply. Then tightly cap the bottle after using.

Orange	12 drops	Vanilla	10 drops
Amyris	8 drops	Amyris	10 drops
Cypress	5 drops	Neroli	6 drops
Lavender	5 drops	Cypress	4 drops

Tangerine	13 drops	Cabreuva	10 drops
Neroli	7 drops	Vanilla	10 drops
Clary Sage	5 drops	Marjoram	5 drops
Guaiacwood	5 drops	Lavender	5 drops

Peace and Calm—Mist Spray

Choose one of these formulas. Fill a fine-mist spray bottle with four ounces (120 ml) of purified water, add the essential oils, tighten the cap, and shake well. Mist numerous times over the head with eyes closed. Breathe the vapors in deeply.

Tangerine	50 drops		Mandarin	60 drops
Amyris	40 drops		Lime	30 drops
Lavender	30 drops		Amyris	30 drops
Cypress	20 drops		Cypress	30 drops
Marjoram	10 drops		Pure Water	4 ounces (120 ml)
Pure Water	4 ounces (120 ml)			

Cabreuva	40 drops		Lime	60 drops
Orange	40 drops		Lavender	30 drops
Spikenard	30 drops		Copaiba	20 drops
Neroli	20 drops		Cypress	20 drops
Marjoram	20 drops		Vanilla	20 drops
Pure Water	4 ounces (120 ml)		Pure Water	4 ounces (120 ml)

Practice Kindness

Goodness exists in each and every one of us. But, when a person lives in a fast-paced and stressful society such as ours, the inundating demands and pressures of everyday life often become overwhelming. And many of our warm, compassionate, kind, and loving feelings can become suppressed, hardly receiving an opportunity to emerge to the surface.

Select one of the *Practice Kindness* application or inhaler formulas. Find a quiet, comfortable place to relax where you will not be disturbed, play soft music (optional), and use the formula. Spend 20–30 minutes thinking about kind deeds to do in order to derive inner satisfaction without expecting anything in return. For example, feed a hungry animal, plant a berry bush to provide food for the birds, go out of your way for a deserving person, or do something special for someone you care about. The acts of kindness should involve giving of yourself and not any material gifts. To help organize your thoughts, fill out the *Practice Kindness Worksheet*.

Practice Kindness—Application

Apply one of these formulas to the upper chest and back of the neck until the oil is fully absorbed into the skin. Breathe the vapors in deeply.

Guaiacwood	4 drops		Spikenard	4 drops
Rose	3 drops		Neroli	3 drops
Pimento Berry	3 drops		Vanilla	3 drops
Carrier Oil	2 teaspoons (10 ml)		Carrier Oil	2 teaspoons (10 ml)

Tangerine	4 drops		Tangerine	4 drops
Sandalwood	3 drops		Spruce	4 drops
Ambrette Seed	3 drops		Helichrysum	2 drops
Carrier Oil	2 teaspoons (10 ml)		Carrier Oil	2 teaspoons (10 ml)

Vanilla	4 drops	Copaiba	4 drops
Guaiacwood	4 drops	Vanilla	3 drops
Rose	2 drops	Gingergrass	3 drops
Carrier Oil	2 teaspoons (10 ml)	Carrier Oil	2 teaspoons (10 ml)

❀

Gingergrass	4 drops	Vanilla	4 drops
Cedarwood (Atlas)	2 drops	Neroli	3 drops
Spearmint	2 drops	Clary Sage	3 drops
Tangerine	2 drops	Carrier Oil	2 teaspoons (10 ml)
Carrier Oil	2 teaspoons (10 ml)		

Practice Kindness—Inhaler

Choose one of these formulas. Combine the essential oils in a small glass bottle with a wide opening. Inhale the vapors slowly and deeply. Then tightly cap the bottle after using.

❀

Champaca Flower	10 drops	Neroli	8 drops
Rose	8 drops	Hyssop Decumbens	8 drops
Guaiacwood	7 drops	Gingergrass	5 drops
Clove Bud	5 drops	Mandarin	5 drops
		Copaiba	4 drops

❀

Lime	10 drops	Vanilla	10 drops
Orange	8 drops	Rose	10 drops
Guaiacwood	5 drops	Neroli	8 drops
Helichrysum	4 drops	Cassia Bark	2 drops
Cassia Bark	3 drops		

❀

Grapefruit	10 drops	Tangerine	10 drops
Vanilla	8 drops	Helichrysum	5 drops
Orange	6 drops	Spruce	5 drops
Cedarwood (Atlas)	3 drops	Havozo Bark	5 drops
Eucalyptus Citriodora	3 drops	Gingergrass	5 drops

❀

Spruce	10 drops	Tangerine	12 drops
Gingergrass	8 drops	Fir Needles	10 drops
Orange	8 drops	Gingergrass	5 drops
Neroli	4 drops	Sandalwood	3 drops

Practice Kindness—Mist Spray

Choose one of these formulas. Fill a fine-mist spray bottle with four ounces (120 ml) of purified water, add the essential oils, tighten the cap, and shake well. Mist numerous times over the head with eyes closed. Breathe the vapors in deeply.

❀ ❀

Tangerine	70 drops	Gingergrass	40 drops
Rose	35 drops	Neroli	40 drops
Vanilla	25 drops	Vanilla	40 drops
Guaiacwood	20 drops	Lime	30 drops
Pure Water	4 ounces (120 ml)	Pure Water	4 ounces (120 ml)

☙

Litsea Cubeba	60 drops	Neroli	60 drops
Orange	40 drops	Vanilla	50 drops
Lime	40 drops	Havozo Bark	30 drops
Patchouli	10 drops	Guaiacwood	10 drops
Pure Water	4 ounces (120 ml)	Pure Water	4 ounces (120 ml)

Premenstrual Ease

Many women experience great distress during the premenstrual time period. These formulas can help make life a little more bearable.

Premenstrual Ease—Application

Apply one of these formulas to the upper chest, abdomen, and the back of the neck until the oil is fully absorbed into the skin. Breathe the vapors in deeply. For best results, repeat application twice daily until relief is attained.

☙

Neroli	4 drops	Spikenard	4 drops
Vanilla	3 drops	Mandarin	3 drops
Cabreuva	3 drops	Vanilla	3 drops
Carrier Oil	2 teaspoons (10 ml)	Carrier Oil	2 teaspoons (10 ml)

☙

Sandalwood	4 drops	Rose	3 drops
Geranium	3 drops	Mandarin	3 drops
Fennel (Sweet)	3 drops	Sandalwood	3 drops
Carrier Oil	2 teaspoons (10 ml)	Gingergrass	1 drop
		Carrier Oil	2 teaspoons (10 ml)

☙

Neroli	4 drops	Clary Sage	3 drops
Clary Sage	3 drops	Cypress	3 drops
Guaiacwood	3 drops	Fennel (Sweet)	2 drops
Carrier Oil	2 teaspoons (10 ml)	Vanilla	2 drops
		Carrier Oil	2 teaspoons (10 ml)

Premenstrual Ease—Inhaler

Select one of these formulas. Combine the essential oils in a small glass bottle with a wide opening. Inhale the vapors slowly and deeply. Then tightly cap the bottle and use again whenever necessary.

☙　　　　　　　　　　☙

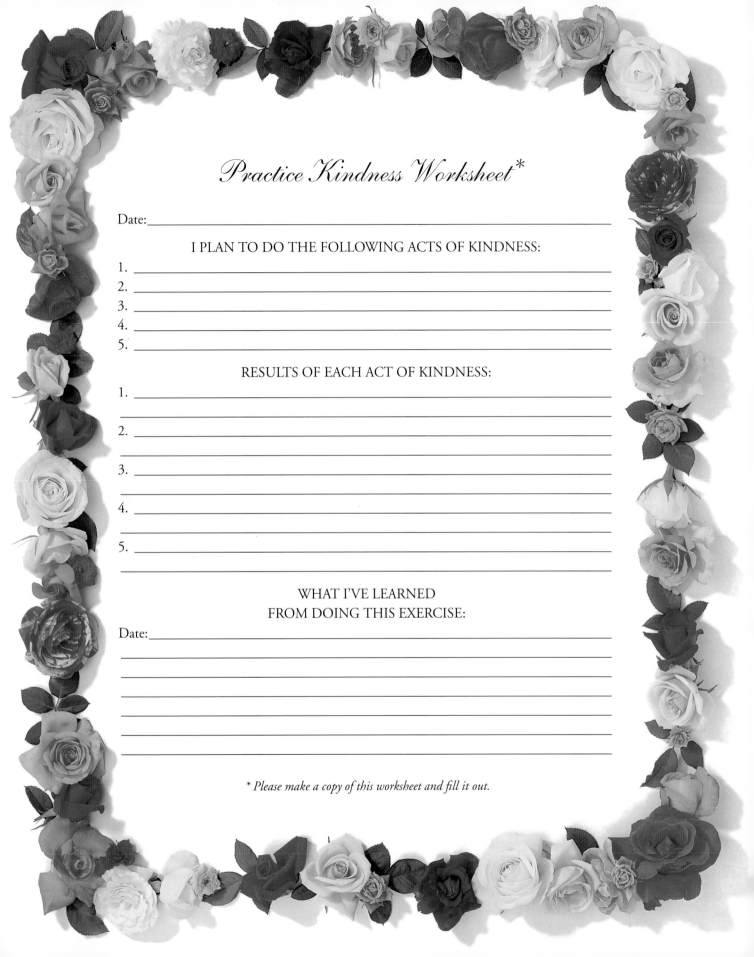

*Practice Kindness Worksheet**

Date:_____

I PLAN TO DO THE FOLLOWING ACTS OF KINDNESS:

1. _____
2. _____
3. _____
4. _____
5. _____

RESULTS OF EACH ACT OF KINDNESS:

1. _____
   _____
2. _____
   _____
3. _____
   _____
4. _____
   _____
5. _____
   _____

WHAT I'VE LEARNED
FROM DOING THIS EXERCISE:

Date:_____
_____
_____
_____
_____
_____
_____

* Please make a copy of this worksheet and fill it out.

Mandarin	15 drops	Sandalwood	10 drops
Neroli	5 drops	Neroli	10 drops
Cedarwood (Atlas)	5 drops	Manuka	5 drops
Vanilla	5 drops	Vanilla	5 drops

Fennel (Sweet)	10 drops	Helichrysum	10 drops
Vanilla	10 drops	Mandarin	10 drops
Clove Bud	5 drops	Rose	7 drops
Spearmint	5 drops	Clove Bud	3 drops

Premenstrual Ease—Mist Spray

Select one of these formulas. Fill a fine-mist spray bottle with two ounces (60 ml) of purified water, add the essential oils, tighten the cap, and shake well. Mist numerous times over the head with eyes closed. Breathe the vapors in deeply.

Fennel (Sweet)	25 drops	Lemon	20 drops
Helichrysum	25 drops	Mandarin	20 drops
Sandalwood	15 drops	Guaiacwood	20 drops
Vanilla	10 drops	Neroli	15 drops
Pure Water	2 ounces (60 ml)	Pure Water	2 ounces (60 ml)

Mandarin	25 drops	Cypress	20 drops
Sandalwood	20 drops	Spikenard	20 drops
Geranium	15 drops	Vanilla	20 drops
Clove Bud	10 drops	Fennel (Sweet)	15 drops
Rose	5 drops	Pure Water	2 ounces (60 ml)
Pure Water	2 ounces (60 ml)		

Orange	25 drops	Tangerine	25 drops
Litsea Cubeba	20 drops	Vanilla	15 drops
Rose	20 drops	Cypress	15 drops
Guaiacwood	10 drops	Neroli	10 drops
Pure Water	2 ounces (60 ml)	Amyris	10 drops
		Pure Water	2 ounces (60 ml)

Recognize Your Treasures

A true state of happiness can only be attained when a person is grateful and appreciative. We shouldn't have to starve in order to appreciate the food we have to eat, become homeless to appreciate our home, or wait until we lose a loved one to realize how precious the person was to us.

Count your blessings. Be grateful for what you have!

Select one of the *Recognize Your Treasures* application or mist spray formulas. Find a quiet, comfortable room to relax where you will not be disturbed, play soft music (optional), and use the formula. Close your eyes and spend 20–30 minutes thinking about everything in your life that you should treasure and all that you have to be thankful for. List them on the *Recognize Your Treasures Worksheet*, then fill out the plan of action. For example, the action plan for appreciating having enough food to eat would be not to be wasteful with food. To treasure the beauty of nature and animals, the action plan would be to take steps that will reduce any polluting and eliminate any harm you are doing to the environment.

Recognize Your Treasures—Application

Apply one of these formulas to the upper chest and the back of the neck until the oil is fully absorbed into the skin. Breathe the vapors in deeply.

Ylang-Ylang	4 drops		Chamomile (Roman)	4 drops
Pimento Berry	3 drops		Vanilla	3 drops
Cedarwood (Atlas)	3 drops		Sandalwood	3 drops
Carrier Oil	2 teaspoons (10 ml)		Carrier Oil	2 teaspoons (10 ml)

Tangerine	4 drops		Vanilla	3 drops
Pimento Berry	2 drops		Guaiacwood	3 drops
Vanilla	2 drops		Spearmint	2 drops
Rose	2 drops		Gingergrass	2 drops
Carrier Oil	2 teaspoons (10 ml)		Carrier Oil	2 teaspoons (10 ml)

Recognize Your Treasures—Mist Spray

Choose one of these formulas. Fill a fine-mist spray bottle with four ounces (120 ml) of purified water, add the essential oils, tighten the cap, and shake well. Mist numerous times over the head with eyes closed. Breathe the vapors in deeply.

Spearmint	40 drops		Tangerine	60 drops
Gingergrass	40 drops		Cedarwood (Atlas)	30 drops
Vanilla	30 drops		Chamomile (Roman)	20 drops
Eucalyptus Citriodora	20 drops		Clove Bud	20 drops
Cedarwood (Atlas)	20 drops		Spearmint	20 drops
Pure Water	4 ounces (120 ml)		Pure Water	4 ounces (120 ml)

Grapefruit	55 drops		Grapefruit	30 drops
Gingergrass	45 drops		Ylang-Ylang	30 drops
Vanilla	25 drops		Lemon	27 drops
Copaiba	10 drops		Vanilla	25 drops
Cypress	10 drops		Helichrysum	25 drops
Cassia Bark	5 drops		Guaiacwood	10 drops
Pure Water	4 ounces (120 ml)		Cassia Bark	3 drops
			Pure Water	4 ounces (120 ml)

*Recognize Your Treasures Worksheet**

Date: _____

TREASURES AROUND ME THAT I NEED TO BE MORE
GRATEFUL AND APPRECIATIVE FOR:

1. _____
2. _____
3. _____
4. _____
5. _____
6. _____
7. _____
8. _____
9. _____
10. _____

PLAN OF ACTION—
I HAVE DECIDED, AFTER DOING THIS EXERCISE, TO MAKE
THESE IMPORTANT CHANGES IN MY LIFE:

_____
_____
_____
_____

RESULTS AFTER 2 MONTHS:

Date: _____
_____
_____
_____

CONCLUSION:

Date: _____
_____
_____
_____

* Please make a copy of this worksheet and fill it out.

Room Air Fragrancing

Bathroom Air Fragrancing—Diffuser

Choose one of these formulas. Place the essential oils in the designated container of the diffuser, then turn on the unit to disperse the aroma into the air.

❧		❧	
Spearmint	50%	Gingergrass	40%
Eucalyptus Citriodora	20%	Litsea Cubeba	30%
Lavender	20%	Lavender	20%
Cassia Bark	10%	Pimento Berry	10%

Bathroom Air Fragrancing—Mist Spray

Choose one of these formulas. Fill a fine-mist spray bottle with four ounces (120 ml) of purified water, add the essential oils, tightly cap the bottle, and shake well. Mist numerous times in the air.

❧		❧	
Cedarwood (Atlas)	60 drops	Peppermint	75 drops
Lemon	60 drops	Cypress	25 drops
Clove Bud	30 drops	Cedarwood (Atlas)	25 drops
Pure Water	4 ounces (120 ml)	Lavender	15 drops
		Cassia Bark	10 drops
		Pure Water	4 ounces (120 ml)

Bedroom Air Fragrancing—Diffuser

Choose one of these formulas. Place the essential oils in the designated container of the diffuser, then turn on the unit to disperse the aroma into the air.

❧		❧	
Tangerine	60%	Lavender	40%
Juniper Berry	20%	Mandarin	40%
Litsea Cubeba	10%	Lemon	20%
Cinnamon Leaf	10%		

Bedroom Air Fragrancing—Mist Spray

Choose one of these formulas. Fill a fine-mist spray bottle with four ounces (120 ml) of purified water, add the essential oils, tightly cap the bottle, and shake well. Mist numerous times in the air.

❧		❧	
Vanilla	50 drops	Tangerine	60 drops
Lemon	50 drops	Lavender	40 drops
Rose	20 drops	Cypress	20 drops
Tangerine	15 drops	Cinnamon Leaf	20 drops
Guaiacwood	15 drops	Marjoram	10 drops
Pure Water	4 ounces (120 ml)	Pure Water	4 ounces (120 ml)

❧   ❧

Dining Room Air Fragrancing—Diffuser

Choose one of these formulas. Place the essential oils in the designated container of the diffuser, then turn on the unit to disperse the aroma into the air.

❂		❂	
Lime	40%	Lemon	40%
Spearmint	30%	Tangerine	30%
Lavender	20%	Cinnamon Leaf	20%
Cinnamon Leaf	10%	Fennel (Sweet)	10%

Dining Room Air Fragrancing—Mist Spray

Choose one of these formulas. Fill a fine-mist spray bottle with four ounces (120 ml) of purified water, add the essential oils, tightly cap the bottle, and shake well. Mist numerous times in the air.

❂		❂	
Gingergrass	60 drops	Spearmint	75 drops
Orange	50 drops	Havozo Bark	30 drops
Litsea Cubeba	30 drops	Cinnamon Leaf	25 drops
Copaiba	10 drops	Copaiba	20 drops
Pure Water	4 ounces (120 ml)	Pure Water	4 ounces (120 ml)

Kitchen Air Fragrancing—Diffuser

Choose one of these formulas. Place the essential oils in the designated container of the diffuser, then turn on the unit to disperse the aroma into the air.

❂		❂	
Tangerine	40%	Lime	50%
Litsea Cubeba	20%	Gingergrass	30%
Grapefruit	20%	Clove Bud	20%
Cassia Bark	10%		
Gingergrass	10%		

Kitchen Air Fragrancing—Mist Spray

Choose one of these formulas. Fill a fine-mist spray bottle with four ounces (120 ml) of purified water, add the essential oils, tightly cap the bottle, and shake well. Mist numerous times in the air.

❂		❂	
Cedarwood (Atlas)	60 drops	Lemon	70 drops
Grapefruit	35 drops	Clove Bud	20 drops
Gingergrass	20 drops	Patchouli	20 drops
Litsea Cubeba	20 drops	Grapefruit	20 drops
Cassia Bark	15 drops	Litsea Cubeba	20 drops
Pure Water	4 ounces (120 ml)	Pure Water	4 ounces (120 ml)

Living Room Air Fragrancing—Diffuser

Choose one of these formulas. Place the essential oils in the designated container of the diffuser, then turn on the unit to disperse the aroma into the air.

❂		❂	
Peppermint	40%	Spearmint	50%
Spearmint	40%	Spruce	30%
Lavender	10%	Eucalyptus Citriodora	20%
Cassia Bark	10%		

Living Room Air Fragrancing—Mist Spray

Choose one of these formulas. Fill a fine-mist spray bottle with four ounces (120 ml) of purified water, add the essential oils, tightly cap the bottle, and shake well. Mist numerous times in the air.

❂		❂	
Grapefruit	50 drops	Spearmint	75 drops
Lime	45 drops	Spruce	40 drops
Vanilla	30 drops	Cinnamon Leaf	25 drops
Copaiba	10 drops	Guaiacwood	10 drops
Hyssop Decumbens	10 drops	Pure Water	4 ounces (120 ml)
Cassia Bark	5 drops		
Pure Water	4 ounces		

Office/Workroom Air Fragrancing—Diffuser

Choose one of these formulas. Place the essential oils in the designated container of the diffuser, then turn on the unit to disperse the aroma into the air.

❂		❂	
Tangerine	40%	Lime	40%
Lemon	30%	Spruce	40%
Peppermint	20%	Grapefruit	20%
Grapefruit	10%		

Office/Workroom Air Fragrancing—Mist Spray

Choose one of these formulas. Fill a fine-mist spray bottle with four ounces (120 ml) of purified water, add the essential oils, tightly cap the bottle, and shake well. Mist numerous times in the air.

❂		❂	
Peppermint	60 drops	Spearmint	65 drops
Lime	35 drops	Lavender	30 drops
Gingergrass	20 drops	Grapefruit	30 drops
Cassia Bark	15 drops	Helichyrsum	25 drops
Copaiba	10 drops	Pure Water	4 ounces (120 ml)
Rosemary	10 drops		
Pure Water	4 ounces (120 ml)		

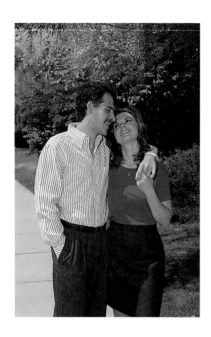

Savor These Precious Moments

The time passes so quickly when you are with someone you care for. Enjoy this special time to the fullest. If you don't have another person to be with, apply the formula on yourself and be your own best friend for this period of time.

Savor These Precious Moments—Massage

Massage one of these formulas into the upper chest, abdomen, back of the neck, and back until the oil is fully absorbed into the skin.

Tangerine	5 drops	Neroli	4 drops
Grapefruit	3 drops	Vanilla	4 drops
Clary Sage	3 drops	Champaca Flower	3 drops
Amyris	2 drops	Gingergrass	3 drops
Spearmint	2 drops	Cedarwood (Atlas)	1 drop
Carrier Oil 1 tablespoon (15 ml)		Carrier Oil 1 tablespoon (15 ml)	

Litsea Cubeba	4 drops	Mandarin	5 drops
Tangerine	4 drops	Chamomile (Roman)	3 drops
Patchouli	3 drops	Neroli	3 drops
Hyssop Decumbens	2 drops	Spearmint	2 drops
Spearmint	2 drops	Spikenard	2 drops
Carrier Oil 1 tablespoon (15 ml)		Carrier Oil 1 tablespoon (15 ml)	

Stop Procrastination

Many of us have chores and work projects that need to get done, but for one reason or another we haven't completed them. When a person procrastinates, it can cause great anxiety to other people who depend on the job getting done. When you've decided that it's time to accomplish the work that you've put off, fill out the *Stop Procrastination Worksheet* and use one of the *Stop Procrastination* massage or mist spray formulas to help make your task more pleasant. Then proceed on with your project.

Stop Procrastination—Massage

Massage one of these formulas into the back of neck, shoulders, upper chest, and abdominal area until the oil is fully absorbed into the skin.

Peppermint	5 drops	Spearmint	5 drops
Fennel (Sweet)	4 drops	Vanilla	4 drops
Sandalwood	3 drops	Litsea Cubeba	3 drops
Thyme	3 drops	Rosemary	3 drops
Carrier Oil 1 tablespoon (15 ml)		Carrier Oil 1 tablespoon (15 ml)	

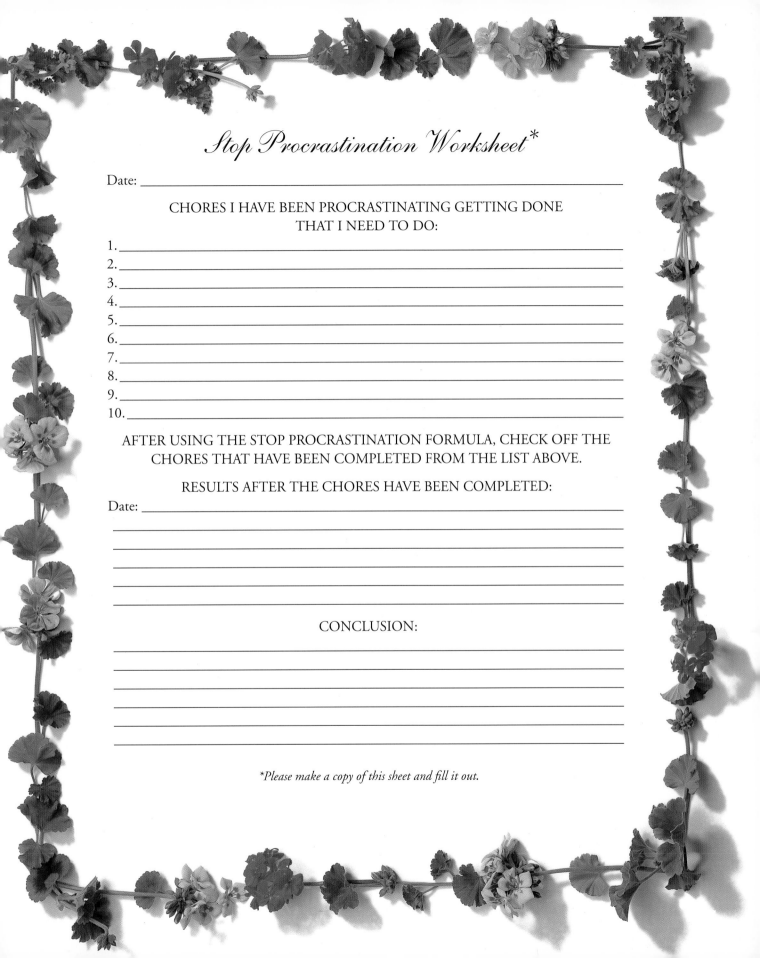

Stop Procrastination Worksheet*

Date: _____

CHORES I HAVE BEEN PROCRASTINATING GETTING DONE THAT I NEED TO DO:

1. _____
2. _____
3. _____
4. _____
5. _____
6. _____
7. _____
8. _____
9. _____
10. _____

AFTER USING THE STOP PROCRASTINATION FORMULA, CHECK OFF THE CHORES THAT HAVE BEEN COMPLETED FROM THE LIST ABOVE.

RESULTS AFTER THE CHORES HAVE BEEN COMPLETED:

Date: _____
_____
_____
_____
_____
_____

CONCLUSION:
_____
_____
_____
_____
_____
_____

*Please make a copy of this sheet and fill it out.

Fennel (Sweet)	4 drops	Hyssop Decumbens	4 drops
Hyssop Decumbens	4 drops	Cedarwood (Atlas)	4 drops
Helichrysum	4 drops	Lime	4 drops
Thyme	3 drops	Thyme	3 drops
Carrier Oil	1 tablespoon (15 ml)	Carrier Oil	1 tablespoon (15 ml)

Stop Procrastination—Mist Spray

Choose one of these formulas. Fill a fine-mist spray bottle with four ounces (120 ml) of purified water, add the essential oils, tighten the cap, and shake well. Mist numerous times over the head with eyes closed. Breathe the vapors in deeply.

◉		◉	
Cedarwood (Atlas)	40 drops	Grapefruit	40 drops
Orange	30 drops	Peppermint	30 drops
Hyssop Decumbens	30 drops	Thyme	30 drops
Rosemary	30 drops	Gingergrass	30 drops
Fennel (Sweet)	20 drops	Vanilla	20 drops
Pure Water	4 ounces (120 ml)	Pure Water	4 ounces (120 ml)
◉		◉	
Spearmint	60 drops	Lime	50 drops
Gingergrass	30 drops	Hyssop Decumbens	30 drops
Cedarwood (Atlas)	20 drops	Thyme	20 drops
Fir Needles	15 drops	Vanilla	20 drops
Cassia Bark	15 drops	Clove Bud	20 drops
Rosemary	10 drops	Patchouli	10 drops
Pure Water	4 ounces (120 ml)	Pure Water	4 ounces (120 ml)

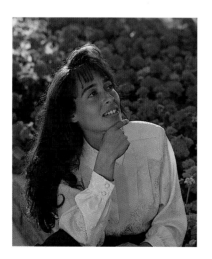

Think Positive Thoughts

We are today a product of our past thoughts, which influenced us to make the decisions we made and led us to take the actions we took. The same holds true now. The thoughts we have today will determine the decisions and actions that will shape our life in future years. It is important for us to promote positive thoughts to help brighten our outlook for the years ahead.

Select one of the *Think Positive Thoughts* application, aroma lamp, diffuser, inhaler, or mist spray formulas. Find a quiet, comfortable place where you will not be disturbed, play soft music (optional), and use the formula. Close your eyes and spend 20–30 minutes allowing yourself to be surrounded with positive energy. Think of the positive actions you need to take to improve your life. Record your thoughts and results on the *Think Positive Thoughts Worksheet*. Place this sheet where it is easily visible so that you can often refer to it. Repeat this exercise three times for the first week, then as often as you feel necessary.

Think Positive Thoughts—Application

Apply one of these formulas to the upper chest and back of the neck until the oil is fully absorbed into the skin. Breathe the vapors in deeply.

❂		❂	
Vanilla	3 drops	Spearmint	4 drops
Spikenard	3 drops	Sandalwood	3 drops
Gingergrass	2 drops	Vanilla	3 drops
Cedarwood (Atlas)	2 drops	Carrier Oil	2 teaspoons (10 ml)
Carrier Oil	2 teaspoons (10 ml)		

❂		❂	
Orange	4 drops	Spruce	3 drops
Cedarwood (Atlas)	4 drops	Vanilla	3 drops
Spruce	2 drops	Litsea Cubeba	2 drops
Carrier Oil	2 teaspoons (10 ml)	Thyme	2 drops
		Carrier Oil	2 teaspoons (10 ml)

❂		❂	
Tangerine	3 drops	Rose	3 drops
Cedarwood (Atlas)	3 drops	Spikenard	3 drops
Thyme	2 drops	Sandalwood	2 drops
Vanilla	2 drops	Lemon	2 drops
Carrier Oil	2 teaspoons (10 ml)	Carrier Oil	2 teaspoons (10 ml)

Think Positive Thoughts—Aroma Lamp

Choose one of these formulas. Fill the container with water, add the essential oils, and heat. Breathe the vapors in deeply.

❂		❂	
Spearmint	15 drops	Tangerine	15 drops
Cedarwood (Atlas)	10 drops	Cedarwood (Atlas)	5 drops
Vanilla	5 drops	Thyme	5 drops
		Vanilla	5 drops

❂		❂	
Orange	10 drops	Litsea Cubeba	10 drops
Thyme	10 drops	Tangerine	10 drops
Spearmint	10 drops	Gingergrass	5 drops
		Cassia Bark	5 drops

❂		❂	
Spearmint	15 drops	Cedarwood (Atlas)	10 drops
Spruce	5 drops	Vanilla	10 drops
Cassia Bark	5 drops	Thyme	5 drops
Cedarwood (Atlas)	5 drops	Cassia Bark	5 drops

Think Positive Thoughts—Diffuser

Choose one of these formulas. Place the essential oils into the designated container of the diffuser, then turn on the unit to disperse the aroma into the air. Breathe the vapors in deeply.

❂	❂

Tangerine	40%	Spearmint	30%
Spearmint	30%	Gingergrass	30%
Fir Needles	20%	Eucalyptus Citriodora	30%
Cassia Bark	10%	Thyme	10%

❂

Spruce	30%	Orange	50%
Orange	30%	Thyme	20%
Grapefruit	30%	Fir Needles	20%
Thyme	10%	Cassia Bark	10%

Think Positive Thoughts—Inhaler

Choose one of these formulas. Combine the essential oils in a small glass bottle with a wide opening. Inhale the vapors slowly and deeply. Then tightly cap the bottle after using.

❂

Spearmint	15 drops	Grapefruit	10 drops
Sandalwood	5 drops	Vanilla	5 drops
Vanilla	5 drops	Clove Bud	5 drops
		Orange	5 drops

❂

Spruce	10 drops	Cedarwood (Atlas)	8 drops
Spearmint	10 drops	Gingergrass	7 drops
Cedarwood (Atlas)	3 drops	Vanilla	5 drops
Cassia Bark	2 drops	Spearmint	5 drops

❂

Tangerine	10 drops	Cedarwood (Atlas)	10 drops
Rose	7 drops	Spearmint	5 drops
Guaiacwood	5 drops	Thyme	5 drops
Vanilla	3 drops	Orange	5 drops

Think Positive Thoughts—Mist Spray

Choose one of these formulas. Fill a fine-mist spray bottle with four ounces (120 ml) of purified water, add the essential oils, tighten the cap, and shake well. Mist numerous times over the head with eyes closed. Breathe the vapors in deeply.

❂

Lemon	50 drops	Spearmint	60 drops
Orange	35 drops	Eucalyptus Citriodora	40 drops
Cedarwood (Atlas)	30 drops	Vanilla	25 drops
Eucalyptus Citriodora	25 drops	Cedarwood (Atlas)	25 drops
Cassia Bark	10 drops	Pure Water	4 ounces (120 ml)
Pure Water	4 ounces (120 ml)		

❂

Think Positive Thoughts Worksheet[*]

Date: _____

LIST SITUATIONS THAT YOU ARE IN THAT YOU MAY BE ABLE TO IMPROVE BY THINKING AND ACTING MORE POSITIVE:

1. _____
2. _____
3. _____
4. _____
5. _____
6. _____

POSITIVE THOUGHTS FOR EACH SITUATION:

1. _____
2. _____
3. _____
4. _____
5. _____
6. _____

POSITIVE ACTIONS TO TAKE:

1. _____
2. _____
3. _____
4. _____
5. _____
6. _____

3-MONTH RESULTS:
HOW HAVE THE CHANGES IMPROVED MY LIFE?

Date: _____

_____

_____

CONCLUSION:

_____

* Please make a copy of this worksheet and fill it out.

Spearmint	50 drops	Tangerine	50 drops
Gingergrass	40 drops	Cedarwood (Atlas)	30 drops
Sandalwood	40 drops	Gingergrass	25 drops
Thyme	20 drops	Litsea Cubeba	25 drops
Pure Water	4 ounces (120 ml)	Vanilla	20 drops
		Pure Water	4 ounces (120 ml)

❧

Vanilla	50 drops	Fir Needles	40 drops
Manuka	30 drops	Orange	40 drops
Havozo Bark	25 drops	Spruce	25 drops
Myrtle	25 drops	Vanilla	25 drops
Mandarin	20 drops	Guaiacwood	20 drops
Pure Water	4 ounces (120 ml)	Pure Water	4 ounces (120 ml)

Wake Up to a Great Day!

It is so important to wake up feeling refreshed, rejuvenated, and in a positive state, ready to have a great day. Select and use one of the diffuser or mist spray formulas and get your day started right!

Wake Up to a Great Day!—Diffuser

Before going to bed, choose one of these formulas. Place the essential oils in the designated container of the diffuser. Set an electric timer to turn on the diffuser ten minutes before your alarm clock rings. Connect the diffuser to the timer and in the morning the reviving aroma will disperse into the air.

❧

Spearmint	50%	Spearmint	50%
Eucalyptus Citriodora	30%	Gingergrass	40%
Cassia Bark	10%	Grapefruit	10%
Thyme	10%		

❧

Spearmint	40%	Grapefruit	40%
Fir Needles	30%	Hyssop Decumbens	30%
Spruce	20%	Lemon	20%
Tangerine	10%	Clove Bud	10%

❧

Hyssop Decumbens	30%	Peppermint	40%
Lime	30%	Rosemary	30%
Gingergrass	20%	Tangerine	30%
Cassia Bark	10%		
Peppermint	10%		

❧

Spearmint	40%	Lime	25%
Lemon	30%	Eucalyptus Citriodora	25%
Spruce	30%	Grapefruit	25%
		Peppermint	25%

Wake Up to a Great Day!—Mist Spray

Select one of these formulas. Fill a fine-mist spray bottle with four ounces (120 ml) of purified water, add the essential oils, tighten the cap, and shake well. Mist numerous times over the head with eyes closed. Breathe the vapors in deeply.

❧

Spearmint	50 drops	Grapefruit	50 drops
Eucalyptus Citriodora	50 drops	Vanilla	30 drops
Vanilla	30 drops	Helichrysum	30 drops
Patchouli	10 drops	Thyme	20 drops
Cassia Bark	10 drops	Clove Bud	20 drops
Pure Water	4 ounces (120 ml)	Pure Water	4 ounces (120 ml)

❧

Lime	50 drops	Grapefruit	60 drops
Peppermint	50 drops	Tangerine	45 drops
Cinnamon Leaf	20 drops	Rose	15 drops
Grapefruit	15 drops	Vanilla	15 drops
Rosemary	15 drops	Guaiacwood	15 drops
Pure Water	4 ounces (120 ml)	Pure Water	4 ounces (120 ml)

Massage

Massage is the oldest and one of the most effective forms of therapy. Its healing power was even known back in ancient times. Hippocrates, the father of medicine, wrote about the importance of massage.

In the Western world, the general public has only in recent years started to realize the healing power and health benefits of touch. A study conducted in 1985 at the University of Miami School of Medicine clearly showed how touch significantly affects the developmental stages of infants. Premature babies were given a 45-minute massage daily. Within ten days these newborns showed a 47% greater improvement in weight, developed more mature behavior and motor skills, and were able to be released six days earlier than the nonmassaged nursery control group.

Enjoying touch is one of the ways to experience a state of worthiness and well-being. Touching is one of the simplest ways to convey and receive feelings of compassion, warmth, closeness, and love.

Exchanging aromatherapy massages with friends and loved ones can help us not only feel great but also satisfy our vital need for touch.

Aches and Pains

Massage one of these formulas into the specific area(s) for 30 minutes and until the oil is fully absorbed into the skin.

❂		❂	
Peppermint	5 drops	Manuka	5 drops
Cabreuva	5 drops	Pimento Berry	4 drops
Thyme	3 drops	Gingergrass	4 drops
Gingergrass	2 drops	Rosemary	2 drops
Carrier Oil	1 tablespoon (15 ml)	Carrier Oil	1 tablespoon (15 ml)

❂		❂	
Havozo Bark	4 drops	Spearmint	4 drops
Cabreuva	4 drops	Manuka	4 drops
Ravensara Aromatica	4 drops	Clary Sage	4 drops
Cinnamon Leaf	3 drops	Lavender	3 drops
Carrier Oil	1 tablespoon (15 ml)	Carrier Oil	1 tablespoon (15 ml)

❂		❂	
Sage (Spanish)	4 drops	Helichrysum	4 drops
Cabreuva	4 drops	Gingergrass	4 drops
Hyssop Decumbens	4 drops	Manuka	4 drops
Fennel (Sweet)	3 drops	Ylang-Ylang	3 drops
Carrier Oil	1 tablespoon (15 ml)	Carrier Oil	1 tablespoon (15 ml)

Back Rub

Massage one of these formulas into the back until the oil is fully absorbed into the skin.

❂		❂	
Cabreuva	4 drops	Gingergrass	5 drops
Geranium	4 drops	Marjoram	4 drops
Peppermint	3 drops	Thyme	3 drops
Pimento Berry	3 drops	Havozo Bark	3 drops
Carrier Oil	1 tablespoon (15 ml)	Carrier Oil	1 tablespoon (15 ml)

❂		❂	
Helichrysum	4 drops	Havozo Bark	4 drops
Spearmint	4 drops	Myrtle	4 drops
Thyme	4 drops	Rosemary	3 drops
Sage (Spanish)	3 drops	Pimento Berry	2 drops
Carrier Oil	1 tablespoon (15 ml)	Cinnamon Leaf	2 drops
		Carrier Oil	1 tablespoon (15 ml)

Chest Rub

Massage one of these formulas into the upper chest and back of the neck until the oil is fully absorbed into the skin. Breathe the vapors in deeply.

❂   ❂

Spruce	5 drops	Ravensara Aromatica	4 drops
Marjoram	4 drops	Gingergrass	4 drops
Thyme	3 drops	Pimento Berry	3 drops
Fennel (Sweet)	3 drops	Helichrysum	2 drops
Carrier Oil 1 tablespoon (15 ml)		Spearmint	2 drops
		Carrier Oil 1 tablespoon (15 ml)	

❂   ❂

Lavender	4 drops	Gingergrass	5 drops
Peppermint	4 drops	Ravensara Aromatica	4 drops
Marjoram	4 drops	Manuka	3 drops
Thyme	3 drops	Marjoram	3 drops
Carrier Oil 1 tablespoon (15 ml)		Carrier Oil 1 tablespoon (15 ml)	

Foot Rejuvenator

Fill a basin with water as warm as you like, add ½ cup (113.4 gm) of epsom salt, and soak feet for 15 minutes. Wipe dry, and massage one of these formulas into the bottoms of the feet, ankles, and calves until the oil is fully absorbed into the skin.

❂   ❂

Spearmint	4 drops	Gingergrass	4 drops
Patchouli	3 drops	Thyme	3 drops
Helichrysum	3 drops	Helichrysum	3 drops
Carrier Oil 2 teaspoons (10 ml)		Carrier Oil 2 teaspoons (10 ml)	

❂   ❂

Helichrysum	4 drops	Peppermint	4 drops
Fir Needles	2 drops	Rosemary	4 drops
Eucalyptus Citriodora	2 drops	Cinnamon Leaf	2 drops
Lime	2 drops	Carrier Oil 2 teaspoons (10 ml)	
Carrier Oil 2 teaspoons (10 ml)			

❂   ❂

Spearmint	4 drops	Litsea Cubeba	4 drops
Cabreuva	4 drops	Rosemary	3 drops
Eucalyptus Citriodora	2 drops	Cabreuva	3 drops
Carrier Oil 2 teaspoons (10 ml)		Carrier Oil 2 teaspoons (10 ml)	

Menstrual and Menopause Comfort

Massage one of these formulas into the upper chest, abdominal area, and lower back until the oil is fully absorbed into the skin. It may be necessary to repeat the application of the formula several times in order to obtain best results.

❂   ❂

Geranium	4 drops	Chamomile (Roman)	4 drops
Helichrysum	4 drops	Fennel (Sweet)	4 drops
Havozo Bark	4 drops	Cypress	4 drops
Clary Sage	3 drops	Rose	3 drops
Almond (Sweet)	2 teaspoons (10 ml)	Almond (Sweet)	2 teaspoons (10 ml)
Evening Primrose	1 teaspoon (5 ml)	Evening Primrose	1 teaspoon (5 ml)

❀

Manuka	4 drops	Geranium	4 drops
Helichrysum	4 drops	Chamomile (Roman)	4 drops
Fennel (Sweet)	4 drops	Neroli	4 drops
Sage (Spanish)	3 drops	Juniper Berry	3 drops
Almond (Sweet)	2 teaspoons (10 ml)	Almond (Sweet)	2 teaspoons (10 ml)
Evening Primrose	1 teaspoon (5 ml)	Evening Primrose	1 teaspoon (5 ml)

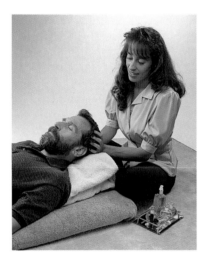

Scalp Massage Before Bedtime

Massage one of these formulas into the scalp before bedtime to promote a restful sleep.

❀		❀	
Spikenard	3 drops	Neroli	4 drops
Neroli	3 drops	Marjoram	3 drops
Orange	2 drops	Clary Sage	3 drops
Vanilla	2 drops	Carrier Oil	2 teaspoons (10 ml)
Carrier Oil	2 teaspoons (10 ml)		

❀		❀	
Chamomile (Roman)	4 drops	Vanilla	4 drops
Tangerine	3 drops	Clary Sage	3 drops
Lavender	3 drops	Spikenard	3 drops
Carrier Oil	2 teaspoons (10 ml)	Carrier Oil	2 teaspoons (10 ml)

❀		❀	
Guaiacwood	4 drops	Vanilla	4 drops
Amyris	3 drops	Manuka	3 drops
Tangerine	3 drops	Lemon	3 drops
Carrier Oil	2 teaspoons (10 ml)	Carrier Oil	2 teaspoons (10 ml)

Soothe Nervous Tension

Massage one of these formulas into the abdominal area, upper chest, back of the neck, shoulders, and back until the oil is fully absorbed into the skin. Breathe the vapors in deeply.

❀   ❀

Spikenard	4 drops	Cypress	4 drops
Chamomile (Roman)	4 drops	Copaiba	4 drops
Vanilla	4 drops	Guaiacwood	4 drops
Sandalwood	3 drops	Clary Sage	3 drops
Carrier Oil 1 tablespoon (15 ml)		Carrier Oil 1 tablespoon (15 ml)	

❀

Neroli	4 drops	Vanilla	4 drops
Tangerine	4 drops	Manuka	4 drops
Cabreuva	4 drops	Cabreuva	4 drops
Juniper Berry	3 drops	Marjoram	3 drops
Carrier Oil 1 tablespoon (15 ml)		Carrier Oil 1 tablespoon (15 ml)	

Stress-Free Feet

Fill a basin with water as warm as you like, add ½ cup (113.4 gm) of epsom salt, and soak feet for 15 minutes. Wipe dry, then massage one of these formulas into the bottoms of the feet, ankles, and calves until the oil is fully absorbed into the skin.

❀

Neroli	5 drops	Amyris	4 drops
Mandarin	5 drops	Lavender	4 drops
Guaiacwood	5 drops	Grapefruit	4 drops
Carrier Oil 1 tablespoon (15 ml)		Ravensara Aromatica	3 drops
		Carrier Oil 1 tablespoon (15 ml)	

❀

Cabreuva	4 drops	Chamomile (Roman)	4 drops
Neroli	4 drops	Lemon	3 drops
Chamomile (Roman)	4 drops	Marjoram	3 drops
Marjoram	2 drops	Cabreuva	3 drops
Spearmint	1 drop	Lavender	2 drops
Carrier Oil 1 tablespoon (15 ml)		Carrier Oil 1 tablespoon (15 ml)	

Tummy Rub

Massage one of these formulas into the abdominal area until the oil is fully absorbed into the skin.

❀

Tangerine	4 drops	Chamomile (Roman)	4 drops
Copaiba	3 drops	Grapefruit	3 drops
Eucalyptus Citriodora	3 drops	Thyme	3 drops
Carrier Oil 2 teaspoons (10 ml)		Carrier Oil 2 teaspoons (10 ml)	

❀

Copaiba	4 drops	Manuka	4 drops
Spearmint	3 drops	Clary Sage	3 drops
Marjoram	3 drops	Fennel (Sweet)	3 drops
Carrier Oil 2 teaspoons (10 ml)		Carrier Oil 2 teaspoons (10 ml)	

❀

Helichrysum	4 drops	Gingergrass	4 drops
Gingergrass	3 drops	Fennel (Sweet)	3 drops
Spearmint	3 drops	Cabreuva	3 drops
Carrier Oil	2 teaspoons (10 ml)	Carrier Oil	2 teaspoons (10 ml)

Personal Care Products

It's so enjoyable and easy to produce your own natural everyday personal body care products. It takes minutes to combine all the ingredients together and use. And remember, you will derive great satisfaction to know that you made these natural products yourself.

Body Powder

Body powder is a great way to freshen and fragrance the skin before going out, or after taking a bath or shower. Select one of these formulas. Measure the amount of arrowroot powder and pour into a wide-mouthed glass jar or a spice powder container; add the essential oils and mix well. Tighten the cap and let the body powder sit for a day so the vapors can permeate the powder with the scent. Apply a small portion on the skin and store for the next use. Store in a dark, cool place. Cornstarch can be substituted for arrowroot powder.

❧

Orange	30 drops	Orange	20 drops
Neroli	20 drops	Helichrysum	10 drops
Guaiacwood	10 drops	Rose	10 drops
Arrowroot Powder	4 tablespoons (56.7 gm)	Ambrette Seed	10 drops
		Clove Bud	10 drops
		Arrowroot Powder	4 tablespoons (56.7 gm)

❧

Grapefruit	20 drops	Spearmint	25 drops
Vanilla	15 drops	Vanilla	15 drops
Copaiba	15 drops	Gingergrass	10 drops
Clove Bud	10 drops	Guaiacwood	10 drops
Arrowroot Powder	4 tablespoons (56.7 gm)	Arrowroot Powder	4 tablespoons (56.7 gm)

❧

Peppermint	20 drops	Tangerine	30 drops
Vanilla	15 drops	Geranium	15 drops
Helichrysum	15 drops	Cedarwood (Atlas)	10 drops
Ravensara Aromatica	10 drops	Pimento Berry	5 drops
Arrowroot Powder	4 tablespoons (56.7 gm)	Arrowroot Powder	4 tablespoons (56.7 gm)

❧

Orange	20 drops	Vanilla	20 drops
Chamomile (Roman)	15 drops	Mandarin	20 drops
Vanilla	15 drops	Helichrysum	15 drops
Fennel (Sweet)	10 drops	Patchouli	5 drops
Arrowroot Powder	4 tablespoons (56.7 gm)	Arrowroot Powder	4 tablespoons (56.7 gm)

◉

Orange	20 drops	Tangerine	25 drops
Spruce	15 drops	Cedarwood (Atlas)	15 drops
Havozo Bark	15 drops	Sage (Spanish)	10 drops
Fir Needles	10 drops	Fennel (Sweet)	5 drops
Arrowroot Powder	4 tablespoons (56.7 gm)	Vanilla	5 drops
		Arrowroot Powder	4 tablespoons (56.7 gm)

◉

Neroli	20 drops	Spearmint	25 drops
Vanilla	20 drops	Manuka	15 drops
Myrtle	10 drops	Havozo Bark	10 drops
Pimento Berry	5 drops	Gingergrass	10 drops
Cabreuva	5 drops	Arrowroot Powder	4 tablespoons (56.7 gm)
Arrowroot Powder	4 tablespoons (56.7 gm)		

◉

Vanilla	20 drops	Orange	20 drops
Ylang-Ylang	20 drops	Gingergrass	15 drops
Neroli	10 drops	Lime	15 drops
Hyssop Decumbens	10 drops	Litsea Cubeba	10 drops
Arrowroot Powder	4 tablespoons (56.7 gm)	Arrowroot Powder	4 tablespoons (56.7 gm)

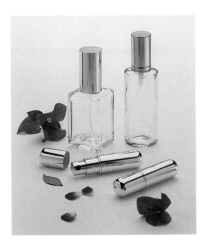

Breath Freshener

Select one of these formulas. Fill a fine-mist spray bottle with two ounces (60 ml) of purified water, add the essential oils, tighten the cap, and shake well. Before using, shake again, and gently mist once or twice directly into the mouth. Enjoy the freshness!

◉

Spearmint	4 drops	Manuka	5 drops
Cinnamon Leaf	4 drops	Helichrysum	5 drops
Orange	2 drops	Pure Water	2 ounces (60 ml)
Pure Water	2 ounces (60 ml)		

◉

Fennel (Sweet)	5 drops	Manuka	5 drops
Orange	3 drops	Tangerine	5 drops
Pimento Berry	2 drops	Pure Water	2 ounces (60 ml)
Pure Water	2 ounces (60 ml)		

◉

Lime	4 drops	Helichrysum	4 drops
Vanilla	3 drops	Vanilla	4 drops
Peppermint	3 drops	Fennel (Sweet)	2 drops
Pure Water	2 ounces (60 ml)	Pure Water	2 ounces (60 ml)

❧

Spearmint	4 drops	Fennel (Sweet)	4 drops
Vanilla	4 drops	Vanilla	3 drops
Clove Bud	2 drops	Orange	3 drops
Pure Water	2 ounces (60 ml)	Pure Water	2 ounces (60 ml)

Douche

Select one of these formulas. Warm the water, then pour into a glass bottle. Add the essential oils and apple cider vinegar, mix well, place into the douche bag, and use.

❧

Geranium	3 drops	Lavender	3 drops
Helichrysum	3 drops	Geranium	3 drops
Ravensara Aromatica	2 drops	Ylang-Ylang	2 drops
Pure Water	16 ounces (480 ml)	Pure Water	16 ounces (480 ml)

❧

Chamomile (Roman)	4 drops	Manuka	3 drops
Sandalwood	4 drops	Rose	3 drops
Pure Water	16 ounces (480 ml)	Cedarwood (Atlas)	2 drops
		Pure Water	16 ounces (480 ml)

❧

Copaiba	3 drops	Neroli	4 drops
Helichrysum	3 drops	Manuka	4 drops
Orange	2 drops	Pure Water	16 ounces (480 ml)
Pure Water	16 ounces (480 ml)		

Foot Deodorant

To help keep your feet smelling nice use one of these formulas. First rub in well 20 drops of aloe vera juice to the bottoms of the feet. Then massage in the essential oils until the formula is fully absorbed into the skin. Dry off with arrowroot powder or cornstarch.

❧

Ravensara Aromatica	3 drops	Guaiacwood	3 drops
Spikenard	1 drop	Chamomile (Roman)	1 drop
Vanilla	1 drop	Vanilla	1 drop

❧

Cabreuva	2 drops	Ravensara Aromatica	3 drops
Manuka	2 drops	Guaiacwood	2 drops
Orange	1 drop		

❧

Cabreuva	2 drops	Myrtle	2 drops
Myrtle	2 drops	Guaiacwood	2 drops
Orange	1 drop	Vanilla	1 drop

Foot Powder

Select one of these formulas. Measure the amount of arrowroot powder and pour into a wide-mouthed glass jar or a spice powder container. Add the essential oils and mix well. Tighten the cap and let the foot powder sit for a day. Mix again before using and apply the necessary amount. Cornstarch can be substituted for arrowroot powder.

❧

Manuka	25 drops	Ravensara Aromatica	20 drops
Cypress	10 drops	Orange	20 drops
Cabreuva	10 drops	Eucalyptus Citriodora	10 drops
Litsea Cubeba	10 drops	Juniper Berry	10 drops
Vanilla	5 drops	Arrowroot Powder	4 tablespoons (56.7 gm)
Arrowroot Powder	4 tablespoons (56.7 gm)		

❧

Guaiacwood	20 drops	Manuka	25 drops
Litsea Cubeba	20 drops	Ravensara Aromatica	25 drops
Copaiba	10 drops	Fennel (Sweet)	10 drops
Chamomile (Roman)	10 drops	Arrowroot Powder	4 tablespoons (56.7 gm)
Arrowroot Powder	4 tablespoons (56.7 gm)		

Hair & Scalp Moisterizing Creme

Select one of these formulas. Place the shea butter in a wide-mouthed glass jar and put the jar in a small pot of water. Heat on a low flame. When the butter has melted, add the jojoba oil and stir well. Remove the jar from the heated water and, as the ingredients cool, mix the essential oils in well, and tightly cap the jar. To use: Dampen the hair with water, apply the necessary amount of creme, rub in well into the scalp, then brush or comb the hair. Store in a dark, cool place.

❧

Shea Butter	2 tablespoons (28.35 gm/30 ml)	Shea Butter	2 tablespoons (28.35 gm/30 ml)
Jojoba	1 tablespoon (15ml)	Jojoba	1 tablespoon (15 ml)
Peppermint	20 drops	Spearmint	20 drops
Cedarwood (Atlas)	10 drops	Vanilla	12 drops
Cabreuva	5 drops	Rosemary	8 drops
Neroli	5 drops		

❧ ❧

Shea Butter	2 tablespoons (28.35 gm/30 ml)	Shea Butter	2 tablespoons (28.35 gm/30 ml)
Jojoba	1 tablespoon (15 ml)	Jojoba	1 tablespoon (15 ml)
Neroli	18 drops	Neroli	25 drops
Mandarin	12 drops	Amyris	10 drops
Guaiacwood	10 drops	Peppermint	5 drops

�

Shea Butter	2 tablespoons (28.35 gm/30 ml)	Shea Butter	2 tablespoons (28.35 gm/30 ml)
Jojoba	1 tablespoon (15 ml)	Jojoba	1 tablespoon (15 ml)
Tangerine	25 drops	Sandalwood	15 drops
Neroli	10 drops	Rose	15 drops
Cedarwood (Atlas)	5 drops	Geranium	10 drops

ⓕ

Shea Butter	2 tablespoons (28.35 gm/30 ml)	Shea Butter	2 tablespoons (28.35 gm/30 ml)
Jojoba	1 tablespoon (15 ml)	Jojoba	1 tablespoon (15 ml)
Ylang-Ylang	10 drops	Spearmint	15 drops
Geranium	10 drops	Amyris	10 drops
Guaiacwood	10 drops	Grapefruit	10 drops
Cedarwood (Atlas)	6 drops	Pimento Berry	5 drops
Pimento Berry	4 drops		

Hair Rinse

To bring out the shine in your hair, rinse with one of these hair formulas. Mix all the ingredients in a glass bottle. Shake well before using. Apply a small portion into the scalp and hair after shampooing. Leave on for about 10–15 minutes and then towel dry. Notice the difference with each washing. Place a label on the bottle and refrigerate after using.

ⓕ

Manuka	5 drops	Sage (Spanish)	5 drops
Spearmint	5 drops	Spruce	5 drops
Cedarwood (Atlas)	4 drops	Spearmint	5 drops
Lavender	3 drops	Copaiba	5 drops
Tangerine	3 drops	Aloe Vera Juice	2 tablespoons (30 ml)
Aloe Vera Juice	2 tablespoons (30 ml)	Apple Cider Vinegar	2 tablespoons (30 ml)
Apple Cider Vinegar	2 tablespoons (30 ml)	Water	28 ounces (840 ml)
Water	28 ounces (840 ml)		

ⓕ

Litsea Cubeba	8 drops		Copaiba	8 drops
Patchouli	7 drops		Cedarwood (Atlas)	5 drops
Chamomile (Roman)	5 drops		Spearmint	5 drops
Aloe Vera Juice	2 tablespoons (30 ml)		Juniper Berry	2 drops
Apple Cider Vinegar	2 tablespoons (30 ml)		Aloe Vera Juice	2 tablespoons (30 ml)
Water	28 ounces (840 ml)		Apple Cider Vinegar	2 tablespoons (30 ml)
			Water	28 ounces (840 ml)

Menstrual Pad Freshener

To help keep you feeling fresh, drop the essential oils onto a menstrual pad and use.

◉			◉	
Manuka	4 drops		Sandalwood	4 drops
Rose	3 drops		Ylang-Ylang	3 drops
◉			◉	
Guaiacwood	4 drops		Manuka	4 drops
Ravensara Aromatica	3 drops		Chamomile (Roman)	3 drops
◉			◉	
Sandalwood	5 drops		Helichrysum	4 drops
Eucalyptus Citriodora	2 drops		Geranium	3 drops
◉			◉	
Vanilla	4 drops		Vanilla	5 drops
Myrtle	3 drops		Copaiba	2 drops
◉			◉	
Lavender	3 drops		Amyris	4 drops
Vanilla	2 drops		Chamomile (Roman)	3 drops
Chamomile (Roman)	2 drops			

Skin Care Cremes

Having healthy-looking skin adds to one's beauty. Try one of these formulas and improve the softness and radiance of your skin. Place the vegetable butter(s) in a wide-mouthed glass jar and put the jar in a small pot of water. Heat on a low flame. When the butter melts, add the carrier oil and stir well. Remove the jar from the heated water and, as the ingredients cool, mix the essential oils in well and tightly cap the jar. Wait several hours until the creme becomes creamy in texture before using. Store in a dark, cool place.

◉ ◉

Cocoa Butter	7 teaspoons	Cocoa Butter	7 teaspoons
	(33.07 gm/35 ml)		(33.07 gm/35 ml)
Shea Butter	3 teaspoons	Shea Butter	3 teaspoons
	(14.17 gm/15 ml)		(14.17 gm/15 ml)
Carrier Oil	6 teaspoons (30 ml)	Carrier Oil	6 teaspoons (30 ml)
Chamomile (Roman)	25 drops	Sandalwood	25 drops
Helichrysum	15 drops	Guaiacwood	15 drops
Cedarwood (Atlas)	10 drops	Havozo Bark	10 drops

ⓔ

Cocoa Butter	7 teaspoons	Cocoa Butter	7 teaspoons
	(33.07 gm/35 ml)		(33.07 gm/35 ml)
Shea Butter	3 teaspoons	Shea Butter	3 teaspoons
	(14.17 gm/15 ml)		(14.17 gm/15 ml)
Carrier Oil	6 teaspoons (30 ml)	Carrier Oil	6 teaspoons (30 ml)
Geranium	20 drops	Spearmint	15 drops
Chamomile (Roman)	20 drops	Vanilla	15 drops
Vanilla	10 drops	Copaiba	15 drops
		Guaiacwood	5 drops

ⓔ

Shea Butter	2 tablespoons	Shea Butter	2 tablespoons
	(28.35 gm/30 ml)		(28.35 gm/30 ml)
Jojoba	8 teaspoons (40 ml)	Jojoba	8 teaspoons (40 ml)
Tangerine	10 drops	Helichrysum	15 drops
Guaiacwood	10 drops	Vanilla	13 drops
Rose	10 drops	Copaiba	12 drops
Cedarwood (Atlas)	10 drops		

ⓔ

Shea Butter	2 tablespoons	Shea Butter	2 tablespoons
	(28.35 gm/30 ml)		(28.35 gm/30 ml)
Jojoba	8 teaspoons (40 ml)	Jojoba	8 teaspoons (40 ml)
Vanilla	24 drops	Spearmint	20 drops
Cedarwood (Atlas)	6 drops	Vanilla	15 drops
Geranium	5 drops	Spruce	5 drops
Ylang-Ylang	5 drops		

Tooth Powder

Make your own natural tooth powder that you can flavor according to your taste preference. Select one of these formulas. Measure the amount of arrowroot powder, pour into a small wide-mouthed glass jar, add the essential oils, stir well, and tightly cap the jar. Let the powder sit for a day. Mix again before using and brush with small amount each time. Store in a dark, cool place.

ⓔ   ⓔ

Manuka	4 drops	Cinnamon Leaf	4 drops
Spearmint	4 drops	Orange	4 drops
Arrowroot Powder	2 tablespoons (28.35 gm)	Arrowroot Powder	2 tablespoons (28.35 gm)

ⓐ

Sage (Spanish)	5 drops	Helichrysum	8 drops
Peppermint	3 drops	Arrowroot Powder	2 tablespoons (28.35 gm)
Arrowroot Powder	2 tablespoons (28.35 gm)		

ⓐ

Geranium	3 drops	Sage (Spanish)	4 drops
Spearmint	3 drops	Helichrysum	4 drops
Helichrysum	2 drops	Arrowroot Powder	2 tablespoons (28.35 gm)
Arrowroot Powder	2 tablespoons (28.35 gm)		

Underarm Deodorant

To help keep you smelling great all day, try one of these formulas. First, apply 10 drops of aloe vera juice to each underarm. Then mix the essential oils in the formula and rub in well into both underarms. Dry any remaining oil residue with a small amount of arrowroot powder or cornstarch, then dab well with a tissue. After a woman shaves her underarms, it is advisable to wait 15 minutes before applying the deodorant to avoid any burning sensation.

Manuka	3 drops	Vanilla	2 drops
Chamomile (Roman)	1 drop	Hibisuc (Ambrette Seed)	2 drops
Neroli	2 drops	Champaca Flower	2 drops
Manuka	2 drops	Vanilla	2 drops
Ravensara Aromatica	2 drops	Champaca Flower	2 drops
Vanilla	2 drops	Orange	1 drop
Myrtle	2 drops	Neroli	2 drops
Vanilla	2 drops	Cabreuva	2 drops

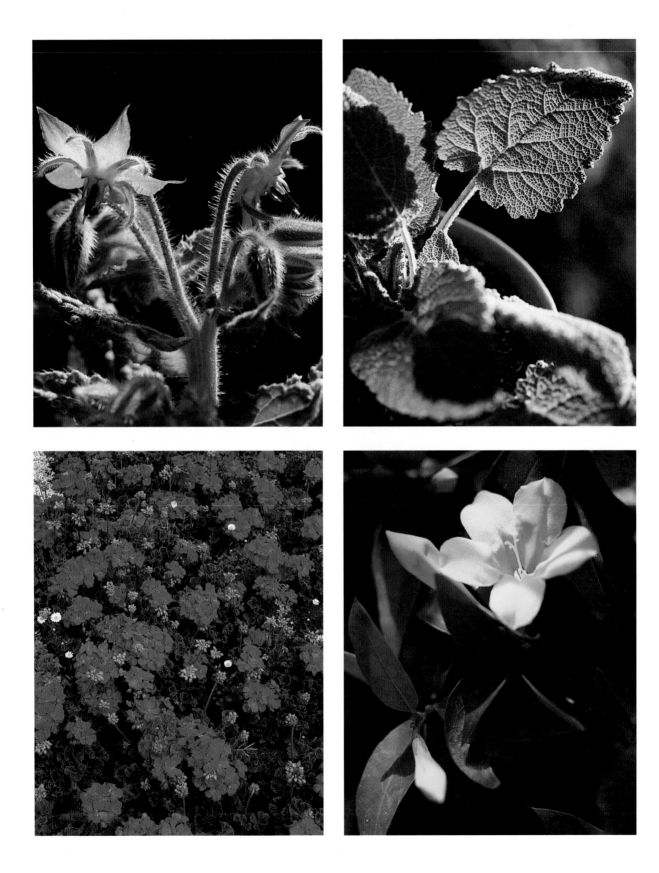

Index

Biography

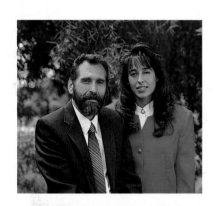

DAVID SCHILLER and CAROL SCHILLER have been instructing aromatherapy classes for colleges as well as other educational organizations since 1989 and formulating essential oil blends since 1986. They are consultants to companies and are the authors of *500 Formulas for Aromatherapy* (Sterling), *Aromatherapy for Mind & Body* (Sterling), *Aromatherapy Oils* (Sterling), and numerous magazine articles. Carol Schiller is also a certified hypnotherapist and graphologist, and instructs classes on these subjects as well.

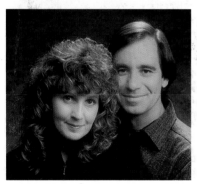

MARVIN and LYNNE CARLTON are the owners of Carltons' Photographic, Inc., in Phoenix, Arizona, started in 1982. Their work has appeared on magazine and book covers and sold in fine art galleries. Both Marvin and Lynne graduated from Brooks Institute of Photography in Santa Barbara, California, in 1978.